# VETERINARY NECROPSY OF DOGS AND CATS

# VETERINARY NECROPSY OF DOGS AND CATS

# CASE BASED APPROACH

Sionagh Smith & Linda Morrison

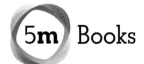

5m Books

First published 2024

Published by

5m Books Ltd,
Lings, Great Easton,
Essex, CM6 2HH, UK
Tel: +44 (0)330 1333 580
www.5mbooks.com

Follow us on
Twitter @5m_Books
Instagram @5m_Books
Facebook @5m_Books
LinkedIn @5m_Books

A catalogue record for this book is available from the British Library.

ISBN 9781789182620
eISBN 9781789183276
DOI 10.52517/9781789183276

Book Layout by Cheshire Typesetting Ltd, Cuddington, Cheshire
Printed by CPI Antony Rowe Ltd, UK
Photos by the suthors unless otherwise indicated
Cover image licensed from Adobe Stock – N. 637124302

# Contents

# Preface: Causes of death in dogs and cats

This book uses real world necropsies of dogs and cats to explore a number of different concepts and practical applications. However, before we begin, we thought it would be of interest to cast our eyes backwards at some of the relevant veterinary literature from the last few decades. Collectively, a number of necropsy surveys have summarised the main causes of death in dogs and cats in different settings and different parts of the world, so we open this book with a brief review of those surveys as a means of 'setting the stage'.

## Causes of death in dogs

The most common causes of death in dogs are neoplasia, old age, trauma, cardiac conditions and behavioural problems.[1,2,3,6,10,13–15,17,20,21] The type of neoplasia often remains unspecified but commonly affected organs include the liver, mammary glands and brain.[1,2] Where specified, lymphoma, haemangiosarcoma and carcinoma are the most frequent types of neoplasia, followed by other forms of sarcoma and central nervous system (CNS) tumours.[1,2,5] Certain breeds commonly reported to be at an overall increased risk of cancer (or at least overrepresented in study populations) are the Afghan Hound, Airedale Terrier, Bernese Mountain Dog, Boxer, Flat-coated Retriever, Golden Retriever, Irish Wolfhound, Leonberger, Rottweiler and Standard Poodle, among others.[1,11] Particular types of tumour also have a tendency to arise in specific breeds: German Shepherd Dogs (GSDs) and Golden Retrievers are prone to haemangiosarcoma,[4,5,8] Boxers to CNS tumours, especially gliomas,[6] and Rottweilers to lymphoma and osteosarcoma.[5,6] A few popular breeds are predisposed to histiocytic sarcoma, including the Golden Retriever, Flat-coated Retriever, Rottweiler and Bernese Mountain Dog.[5,6]

'Old age' is frequently cited as a cause of death (up to approximately 20% of deaths depending on study), but it is often not clearly defined.[1,10,11] Not all surveys are able to confirm whether dogs dying of old age are euthanised or die naturally but it seems likely (and intuitive) that most are euthanised, and a few studies do confirm that the majority of overall deaths are due to euthanasia.[11,14,18] Depending on survey, trauma can account for up to almost 20% of deaths and, where specified, car accidents are the single most common cause;[1,2] this can vary significantly, however. Causes of cardiac-related deaths are often fairly non-specific and inconsistently listed as 'cardiac', 'cardiac failure', 'heart failure', 'unspecified defect or 'heart attack'.[1,10,11,17] Some surveys provide less ambiguous diagnoses, such as cardiomyopathy (including dilated), mitral valve disease, cardiomegaly, endocardiosis, congenital defect and heart murmur.[1,2] The frequency of deaths due to behavioural problems also varies considerably.[11,17,21] The exact behavioural issue is usually not expanded upon, due to the nature of the raw data available, but aggression features in several studies.[14,17,21]

There is also substantial variation in disease terminology and classification across different studies, which makes it difficult to compare directly. However, less commonly reported causes of death comprise neurological diseases (including epilepsy/seizures), locomotor disturbances, renal failure, gastrointestinal disease (e.g. gastric dilatation and volvulus, pancreatitis, foreign body, parvovirus), cerebrovascular accident ('stroke'), septicaemia, hepatic disease and pneumonia.[1,2,14,15,20] Aside from inherited conditions, certain non-neoplastic conditions are more likely in specific breeds, examples including parvovirus enteropathy in Rottweilers[9,15] and GSDs;[9] and gastric dilatation and volvulus in Akitas, Great Danes, Dogues de Bordeaux, GSDs, Irish Setters, Newfoundlands and Weimaraners.[7,16]

Cause of death is not always established, and the rate of 'inconclusives' ranges from approximately 5% to approximately 12% in the studies we reviewed.[1,5,10] Even when necropsy reports are available, the cause of death remains unclear in up to 12% of cases.[5] However, full and complete necropsy, with follow-up histopathology as required, allows for a final and more definitive diagnosis, in contrast to population surveys, which are much more prone to subjectivity and speculation.

Finally, it is worth noting that the most commonly reported causes of death in dogs under the care of first opinion practices are a little different, at least in the UK. Musculoskeletal disorders, inability to stand/collapse, mass-associated disorder, lower respiratory tract disease and neurological conditions feature more prominently.[14,15,17,18] Nonetheless, multiple breed-specific surveys reviewing causes of death in West Highland White Terriers, Greyhounds, GSDs and Rottweilers, still report neoplasia in the top three most frequent causes.[14,15,17,18]

## Causes of death in cats

There are fewer studies recording causes of death in cats and too few to allow broad generalisations. One UK-based questionnaire study of reasons for feline euthanasia listed neoplasia, old age and trauma as most common causes, although urinary disease was also highlighted.[21] The reason for veterinary related euthanasia (as opposed to economic and behavioural reasons) was unstated in up to one-third of reported cases. Another 10-year retrospective survey described trauma as the most common cause (~40% of deaths), with heart disease the second most common (20% of deaths). Intestinal, respiratory and urinary tract disorders also featured significantly, accounting for at least 5% of deaths each. Cause of death was not identified in just over 12% of cats.[12] A Malaysian necropsy survey of 866 cats also reported traumatic injury as the most commonly recorded health problem (19.5% of necropsies). Road traffic accidents were the most common reason, followed by 'high rise syndrome', blunt trauma, fighting and trauma of unknown origin.[20]

## References

1 Adams, V. J., Evans, K. M., Sampson, J., & Wood, J. L. N. (2010). Methods and mortality results of a health survey of purebred dogs in the UK. *Journal of Small Animal Practice*, *51*(10), 512–524. https://doi.org/10.1111/j.1748-5827.2010.00974.x

2 Bonnett, B. N., Egenvall, A., Hedhammar, A., & Olson, P. (2005). Mortality in over 350,000 insured Swedish dogs from 1995–2000: I. Breed-, gender-, age- and cause-specific rates. *Acta Veterinaria Scandinavica*, *46*(3), 105–120. https://doi.org/10.1186/1751-0147-46-105

3 Bronson, R. T. (1982). Variation in age at death of dogs of different sexes and breeds. *American Journal of Veterinary Research*, *43*(11), 2057–2059.

4 Brown, N. O., Patnaik, A. K., & MacEwen, E. G. (1985). Canine hemangiosarcoma: Retrospective analysis of 104 cases. *Journal of the American Veterinary Medical Association*, *186*(1), 56–58.

5 Craig, L. E. (2001). Cause of death in dogs according to breed: A necropsy survey of five breeds. *Journal of the American Animal Hospital Association*, *37*(5), 438–443. https://doi.org/10.5326/15473317-37-5-438

6 Gardner, H. L., Fenger, J. M., & London, C. A. (2016). Dogs as a model for cancer. *Annual Review of Animal Biosciences*, *4*, 199–222. https://doi.org/10.1146/annurev-animal-022114-110911

7 Glickman, L. T., Glickman, N. W., Schellenberg, D. B., Raghavan, M., & Lee, T. L. (2000). Incidence of and breed-related risk factors for gastric dilatation-volvulus in dogs. *Journal of the American Veterinary Medical Association*, *216*(1), 40–45. https://doi.org/10.2460/javma.2000.216.40

8 Holt, D., Van Winkle, T., Schelling, C., & Prymak, C. (1992). Correlation between thoracic radiographs and postmortem findings in dogs with hemangiosarcoma: 77 cases (1984–1989). *Journal of the American Veterinary Medical Association*, *200*(10), 1535–1539.

9 Houston, D. M., Ribble, C. S., & Head, L. L. (1996). Risk factors associated with parvovirus enteritis in dogs: 283 cases (1982–1991). *Journal of the American Veterinary Medical Association*, *208*(4), 542–546.

10 Lewis, T. W., Wiles, B. M., Llewellyn-Zaidi, A. M., Evans, K. M., & O'Neill, D. G. (2018). Longevity and mortality in Kennel Club registered dog breeds in the UK in 2014. *Canine Genetics and Epidemiology*, *5*, 10. https://doi.org/10.1186/s40575-018-0066-8

11 Michell, A. R. (1999). Longevity of British breeds of dog and its relationships with sex, size, cardiovascular variables and disease. *Veterinary Record*, *145*(22), 625–629. https://doi.org/10.1136/vr.145.22.625

12 Olsen, T. F., & Allen, A. L. (2001). Causes of sudden and unexpected death in cats: A 10-year retrospective study. *Canadian Veterinary Journal*, *42*(1), 61–62.

13 O'Neill, D. G., Church, D. B., McGreevy, P. D., Thomson, P. C., & Brodbelt, D. C. (2013). Longevity and mortality of owned dogs in England. *Veterinary Journal*, *198*(3), 638–643. https://doi.org/10.1016/j.tvjl.2013.09.020

14 O'Neill, D. G., Coulson, N. R., Church, D. B., & Brodbelt, D. C. (2017). Demography and disorders of German Shepherd dogs under primary veterinary care in the UK. *Canine Genetics and Epidemiology*, *4*, 7. https://doi.org/10.1186/s40575-017-0046-4

15 O'Neill, D. G., Seah, W. Y., Church, D. B., & Brodbelt, D. C. (2017). Rottweilers under primary veterinary care in the UK: Demography, mortality and disorders. *Canine Genetics and Epidemiology*, *4*, 13. https://doi.org/10.1186/s40575-017-0051-7

16 O'Neill, D. G., Case, J., Boag, A. K., Church, D. B., McGreevy, P. D., Thomson, P. C., & Brodbelt, D. C. (2017). Gastric dilation-volvulus in dogs attending UK emergency-care veterinary practices: Prevalence, risk factors and survival. *Journal of Small Animal Practice*, *58*(11), 629–638. https://doi.org/10.1111/jsap.12723

17 O'Neill, D. G., Ballantyne, Z. F., Hendricks, A., Church, D. B., Brodbelt, D. C., & Pegram, C. (2019). West Highland White Terriers under primary veterinary care in the UK in 2016: Demography, mortality and disorders. *Canine Genetics and Epidemiology*, *6*, 7. https://doi.org/10.1186/s40575-019-0075-2

18 O'Neill, D. G., Rooney, N. J., Brock, C., Church, D. B., Brodbelt, D. C., & Pegram, C. (2019). Greyhounds under general veterinary care in the UK during 2016: Demography and common disorders. *Canine Genetics and Epidemiology*, *6*, 4. https://doi.org/10.1186/s40575-019-0072-5

19 Proschowsky, H. F., Rugbjerg, H., & Ersbøll, A. K. (2003). Mortality of purebred and mixed-breed dogs in Denmark.

*Preventive Veterinary Medicine*, *58*(1–2), 63–74. https://doi.org/10.1016/s0167-5877(03)00010-2

20 Rathiymaler, M., Zamri-Saad, M., & Annas, S. (2017). Disease conditions in cats and dogs diagnosed at the PostMortem Laboratory of the Faculty of Veterinary Medicine, Universiti Putra Malaysia between 2005 and 2015. *Pertanika Journal of Tropical Agricultural Science*, *40*, 389–398.

21 Stead, A. C. (1982). Euthanasia in the dog and cat. *Journal of Small Animal Practice*, *23*(1), 37–43. https://doi.org/10.1111/j.1748-5827.1982.tb01633.x

# Acknowledgements

We sincerely thank our colleagues, friends and past mentors who kindly helped and inspired us in the development of this book; particular thanks to Alistair Cox, Professor Linden Craig, Dr Alexandra Malbon, Dr Steven McOrist, Dr Adrian Philbey, Professor Elspeth Milne, Professor Susan Rhind and Dr David Walker for their contributions (images and/or advice).

Special thanks to our families; those no longer with us are always in our thoughts.

# Abbreviations

| | | | | |
|---|---|---|---|---|
| ACTH | adrenocorticotrophic hormone | | GIT | gastrointestinal tract |
| ALP | alkaline phosphatase | | GMS | Gomori methanamine silver stain |
| ALT | alanine aminotransferase | | GSD | German Shepherd Dog |
| ARDS | acute respiratory distress syndrome | | Hb | haemoglobin |
| AST | aspartate transaminase | | IgA | immunoglobulin A |
| AV | atrioventricular | | IMHA | immune-mediated haemolytic anaemia |
| BOAS | brachycephalic obstructive airway syndrome | | IVDD | intervertebral disc disease |
| CEH | cystic endometrial hyperplasia | | IVS | interventricular septum |
| CK | creatine kinase | | MD | morphological diagnosis |
| CNS | central nervous system | | NBF | neutral buffered formalin |
| COX | cyclooxygenase | | NSAID | non-steroidal anti-inflammatory drug |
| CSF | cerebrospinal fluid | | PCR | polymerase chain reaction |
| CT | computed tomography | | PCV | packed cell volume |
| DIC | disseminated intravascular coagulopathy | | PD | polydipsia |
| DJD | degenerative joint disease | | PPE | personal protection equipment |
| DSD | disorder of sexual development | | PSS | portosystemic shunts |
| FGESF | feline gastrointestinal eosinophilic sclerosing fibroplasia | | PTE | pulmonary artery thromboembolism |
| | | | PTH | parathyroid hormone |
| FIP | feline infectious peritonitis | | PU | polyuria |
| FIV | feline immunodeficiency virus | | RBC | red blood cells |
| GDV | gastric dilation and volvulus | | RCVS | Royal College of Veterinary Surgeons |
| GI | gastrointestinal | | RTA | road traffic accident |
| GIST | gastrointestinal stromal tumour | | TF | tissue factor |

# Introduction

This book takes a case-based approach to examples of canine and feline necropsies. We use the word 'necropsy' as it avoids the debate about how to spell *postmortem*[1] although we recognise terminology preferences vary (but there is literally more than one way to skin a cat). The cases cover most of the main organ systems and our colour coding aims to flag particular topics in each question (e.g. lesion description; pathogenesis; health and safety – see Fig. 1.1). With one or two exceptions, each case has three main questions – although some may be subdivided.

1. Describe any abnormalities.
2. Provide a diagnosis.
3. The third question varies with each case.

Since we are asking you to describe lesions, some lesion description guidelines follow this introduction (when a scale bar appears in an image, the bar equates to 1 cm). Providing a diagnosis is an opportunity to practise creating a morphological diagnosis or an aetiological diagnosis (which you will frequently see in biopsy and necropsy reports). Further explanation regarding the formulation of these diagnoses is also provided below. Throughout animal ages are shortened, e.g. 10Y for 10 year old.

## How to describe a lesion

The approach to describing a lesion is fairly straightforward if you remember the features below, bearing in mind that you do not have to rigidly include each feature for every lesion – some features may not always be apparent. Also see Table 1.1 for examples of terms used in describing lesions.

1. Location
   A beautifully detailed description does not mean very much if you forget to say where it is. Try to be as specific as possible about where in the organ the lesion is, such as the cortex of the kidney, the mucosa of the jejunum, the dorsal aspect of the digit (remembering to include which digit and which paw), the epicardial, myocardial or endocardial surface of the left ventricle (i.e. not simply 'in the heart'), etc. It is also very important to include whether the lesion is restricted to the surface or if it extends into the parenchyma (lesions in the parenchyma are more likely to be pathologically significant as a rule).

2. Distribution (and number) – the main distribution descriptors are:

   a. Focal: The lesion is solitary.
   b. Multifocal: Two or more lesions. If there are many lesions, there is no need to count them all individually. It is sufficient to give an approximation (e.g. between 30–40) or, if there are too many to count, describe as myriad or innumerable.
   c. Multifocal to coalescing: Two or more lesions with more than one lesion touching each other.
   d. Diffuse: Entire organ affected such that you **cannot see** any normal organ tissue. Hepatic fatty change is one of the best examples of this.
   e. Segmental: Very useful for a tubular organ such as the intestine, uterus, ureter or blood vessel.
   f. Others: Descriptors such as *focally extensive* or *regionally extensive* can be helpful if a solitary lesion is quite large or more extensive, but not yet diffuse (perhaps involving more than half of a liver or lung lobe). *Unilateral* and *bilateral* also add informative detail.

- ◼ Practical technique
- ◼ Lesion recognition
- ◼ Common artefacts and pitfalls
- ◻ Prioritisation of findings
- ◼ Approach to difficult cases
- ◻ Generation of pathological differential diagnoses lists
- ◻ Integration of pathological findings with clinical aspects
- ◼ Health and safety
- ◼ Pathogenesis

Fig. 1.1 Case colour coding.

Note that 'miliary' is not a distribution although it often creeps in inappropriately when there is a need to describe multiple, usually small, lesions scattered throughout an organ. Miliary means 'like millet seed' and usually refers to the gritty, granular feeling under the skin of dogs or cats with flea bite dermatitis (miliary dermatitis). It is also used to describe small granulomas in lungs with tuberculosis. It has evolved to be used as a synonym for *multifocal* but this is incorrect; *multifocal* is much more appropriate. If there are myriad small lesions scattered throughout an organ, 'disseminated multifocally' can help to create the image in the mind's eye.

3. Size

When possible, always measure lesions with a ruler but if there is not one available you can estimate sizes if you know your handspan/length of a finger. Most lesions are three dimensional so always try to include height, width and depth, unless it is spherical when a single diameter will be enough. For more extensive lesions, it might make more sense to define the area of the organ affected by the lesion. For example: 'approximately 60% of the right caudal lung lobe is dark red'. It is best to avoid comparison with foodstuffs such as peas and grapes, or other items such as golf balls.

4. Shape

As with size, remember that some shapes do not really work for three dimensional lesions, e.g. circular only applies to a two-dimensional lesion; spherical is better for a three-dimensional lesion. There are shapes that are used a lot, such as spherical, circular, oval and irregular, but a few others are suggested in Table 1.1. This is not an exhaustive list and there is nothing to stop you from using your own imagination!

5. Colour

This can be slightly tricky as we all perceive colours differently and many lesions are a shade of red, grey or tan. However, pathological lesions can cover the rainbow (see Table 1.2). To enhance a colour description there are one or two other terms that can be used, such as shiny or dull (for surfaces of lesions), translucent or opaque (often used for fluids).

6. Borders

How clearly can you see where the lesion starts and stops? Main terms used to describe this feature are well-demarcated or poorly demarcated/ill-defined.

7. Consistency

How does the lesion (or organ) feel when you gently palpate or squeeze it? Firmness might suggest fibrosis (scarring), hard tissue is likely to be ossified or mineralised. If a normally firm organ becomes soft or friable, this might suggest necrosis, but it can also be associated with autolysis. There are examples in Table 1.1.

8. Texture

How does this differ from consistency? Texture relates more to how the lesion feels when you gently run your fingers over its surface. See Table 1.1 and remember you can be creative here too.

NOTE: While consistency and texture can be difficult to evaluate on an image, they are easier to identify when it is your case.

## How to create a morphological diagnosis

A morphological diagnosis (MD) is a diagnosis that is based on the appearance of the organ. It may be used in the macroscopic (gross) or microscopic context and lends itself best to inflamed organs but can be adapted to other processes such as cavity effusions. The MD does not tell us the cause, that is the realm of the aetiological diagnosis (see below). However, the purpose of the MD is to provide a pathological summary of the processes likely to be at play in a diseased organ **and**, more importantly, to assist in drawing up a likely differential diagnosis list, which in turn facilitates ancillary testing aimed at defining the cause.

To create a MD for lesions the following method is used (see Table 1.3):

SEVERITY + DISTRIBUTION + CHRONICITY + [OPTIONAL MODIFIER] + ORGAN

When creating a morphological diagnosis for neoplasms, only the organ and type of neoplasia are required, e.g. gastric lymphoma, cutaneous squamous cell carcinoma, etc.

## Description and morphological diagnosis practice examples

Use Figure 1.2 to practise providing a description and provide a MD for this feline kidney lesion.

### Suggested description

| | |
|---|---|
| Location | Kidney, specifically the parenchyma of the cortex and outer medulla |
| Distribution | Focal (the two lesions are the same lesion halved) |
| Size | Approximately 2 × 1.5 cm (or replacing approximately one-quarter of the kidney) |
| Shape | Reniform! It is oval with an indentation and has a bulging cut surface |
| Colour | White |
| Border | Well-demarcated |
| Consistency | Soft |
| Texture | Smooth |

Table 1.1 Main descriptors in macroscopic pathology.

| Distribution | Shape | Consistency | Texture |
|---|---|---|---|
| Diffuse | Arborising (branching) | Firm | Chalky |
| Focal | Bosselated (covered in multiple protuberances) | Fluctuant | Granular |
| Focally extensive | Botryoid (like a bunch of grapes) | Gelatinous | Greasy |
| Multifocal | Circular | Hard | Gritty |
| Multifocal, coalescing | Crescent, curved | Mucoid (mainly discharges or fluids) | Ridged |
| Regionally extensive | Depressed (below the normal surface) | Rubbery | Rough |
| Segmental | Flush (level with normal surface) | Soft | Slimy |
| | Fungiform (mushroom) | Spongy | Smooth |
| | Irregular | Sticky | |
| | Linear (in a line) | Tacky (e.g. if dehydrated) | |
| | Oval | Turgid | |
| | Reniform (kidney shaped; indented) | Viscous (especially fluids) | |
| | Raised (above the normal surface) | Waxy (e.g. amyloid deposition can confer a waxy texture) | |
| | Rhomboid | | |
| | Serpiginous (linear and irregular, 'like a snake') | | |
| | Spherical | | |
| | Stellate (star shaped) | | |
| | Triangular | | |
| | Umbilicated (centrally depressed) | | |

Full description: Within the parenchyma of the renal cortex and outer medulla there is a focal, white, well-demarcated, reniform, soft, smooth mass that bulges on cut section and measures approximately 1 × 1.5 cm.

## Morphological diagnosis

This is a neoplasm so the MD only needs to comprise (1) the organ and (2) the name of the neoplasm. This is *renal lymphoma* but *renal carcinoma* is a reasonable differential.

Use Figure 1.3 to practise providing a description and provide a MD for this canine abdominal cavity.

## Suggested description

| | |
|---|---|
| Location | Peritoneal cavity |
| Distribution | Diffuse, although mottled |
| Size | This is less applicable for this particular example as the lesion affects multiple serosal surfaces and diffusely involves the peritoneum. However, the description |

could be enhanced by adding a percentage of surface area affected, in this case >80%.

| | |
|---|---|
| Shape | Not applicable here |
| Colour | Dark red to purple |
| Border | Ill-defined |
| Consistency | Not applicable as this lesion is effectively a change in colour. However, some surfaces are a little rougher than normal (e.g. intestinal serosa) |
| Texture | Some surfaces are finely granular (or have a 'ground glass' appearance, notably the small intestinal serosa). |

In addition: the peritoneal cavity contains a moderate amount (at least 30 ml) of red fluid.

Full description: There is virtually diffuse dark red to purple mottling of the peritoneal surface, particularly the intestinal serosa, parietal peritoneum and urinary bladder serosa. The peritoneal cavity also contains at least 30 ml of dark red fluid.

**Table 1.2** Colour descriptors used in in pathology.

| Colour | Potential significance |
| --- | --- |
| Black | Melanin; blood will also become black after fixation. |
| Blue | Not common – may be associated with cyanosis or some bruises. |
| Brown (beige, fawn, tan) | Lots of lesions may be brown from inflammation to necrosis to hepatic fatty change. |
| Green | Most commonly indicates bile staining, but necrosis may be green.  Eosinophil-rich exudates can also be faintly green-tinged; pus is sometimes green. |
| Grey, white, off-white | Necrosis; inflammation; fibrosis too.<br>If the tissue is white and hard it commonly suggests mineralisation or ossification but also cartilaginous lesions. Areas of necrosis (especially fat necrosis), lymphoid lesions (such as lymphoid hyperplasia in lymph nodes, spleen, intestinal Peyer's patches) and areas of fibrosis or fat infiltration may also appear white. |
| Purple | Usually suggests haemorrhage but could occur with haemorrhagic necrosis or in an infarct. |
| Red | Blood – haemorrhage, hyperaemia (in areas of inflammation), congestion. Atelectatic (collapsed) lungs are red due to lack of air (which makes them their normal pink).<br>Necrosis may be red, especially in acute infarcts and ulcers. |
| Yellow (orange) | Most commonly observed with icterus (hyperbilirubinaemia) but pus and fibrin are typically yellow and some necrotic tissue may also appear yellow. |

## Morphological diagnosis

Severe, diffuse, acute peritonitis with moderate serosanguineous peritoneal effusion.

For the above example, it is possible that the effusion is actually frank blood (i.e. sanguineous). The only way to be sure is to evaluate the packed cell volume (PCV).

## Adaptation of the morphological diagnosis to cavity effusions and exudates

The MD approach described above can be adapted to cavity effusions in the following way:

| SEVERITY+ MODIFIER + CAVITY INVOLVED + 'EFFUSION' or 'EXUDATE' |
| --- |

Example 1: 20 ml of red-tinged watery fluid in the pericardial sac of a large breed dog:

| Moderate serosanguineous pericardial effusion |
| --- |

Example 2: 50 ml of pus in the thoracic cavity of a cat:

| Moderate purulent pleural exudate (pyothorax) |
| --- |

## How to create an aetiological diagnosis

The structure is similar to the MD for a neoplasm; all that is required is the affected organ and the aetiological agent.

Example 1: Leptospira infection of the liver

| Hepatic leptospirosis (or leptospiral hepatitis is acceptable) |
| --- |

Example 2: Toxin-induced necrosis in the kidney

| Toxic nephropathy (renal toxicosis) |
| --- |

## Necropsy and tissue sampling: general guidelines

### To necropsy or not to necropsy

1. For those working in a pathology department or similar, the decision is made for you.
2. For those working in practice, consider the following before going ahead.

   a. Are there any potential legal ramifications or are any external welfare or prosecuting authorities involved, such as police? If so, it is strongly advisable to send the animal for an independent necropsy. If this is not possible for reasons such as geography, transport or weather-related limitations, at least speak to a veterinary pathologist before proceeding.
   b. Are there any health and safety risks?

3. Either way, always seek permission from the owner, including signed consent.

Table 1.3.  Construction of a morphological diagnosis.

| Severity | Distribution | Chronicity* | Modifier† | Organ | | |
| --- | --- | --- | --- | --- | --- | --- |
| | | | | Example organ | Inflamed (-itis) | Diseased (-opathy)†† |
| Minimal | Diffuse | Peracute (hours) | Bilateral | Brain | Encephalitis | Encephalopathy (e.g. hepatic encephalopathy) |
| Mild | Focal | Acute (a few days) | Fibrinous | Kidney | Nephritis | Nephropathy |
| Moderate | Focally extensive | Subacute (up to a week) | Granulomatous | Liver | Hepatitis | Hepatopathy |
| Severe | Multifocal | Chronic (more than a week) | Haemorrhagic | Lung | Pneumonia (or pneumonitis) | – |
| | Multifocal - coalescing | Chronic active (evidence of chronic inflammation with ongoing active component e.g. due to self-trauma of non-healing wound) | Necrotising | Myocardium | Myocarditis | Cardiomyopathy |
| | Regionally extensive | | Pyogranulomatous | Skin | Dermatitis | Dermatopathy |
| | Segmental | | Suppurative (purulent) | Small intestine | Enteritis | Enteropathy |
| | | | Unilateral | Testis | Orchitis | Orchiopathy is technically correct but is infrequently used in practice! |

Notes: *How old is the lesion? This category is very subjective and somewhat arbitrary. † The modifier typically further classifies an inflammatory exudate but other features can be considered as modifiers (e.g. transmural, mural, unilateral, etc). †† '-opathy' used as a suffix implies that an organ is diseased but it is a very general and non-specific term.

NB: A lesion is best considered chronic when there is evidence of tissue loss or tissue repair/fibrosis.

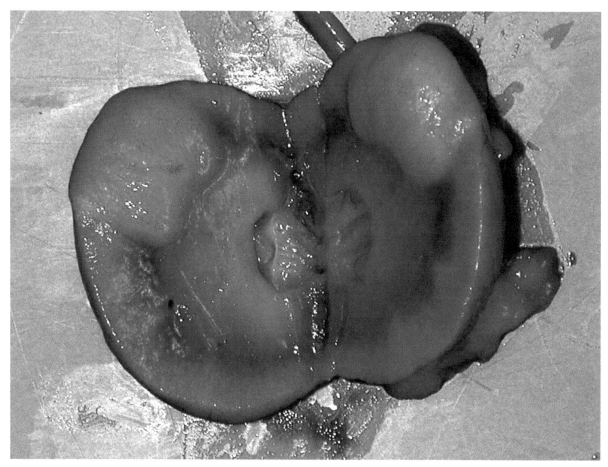

Fig. 1.2 Practice example 1.

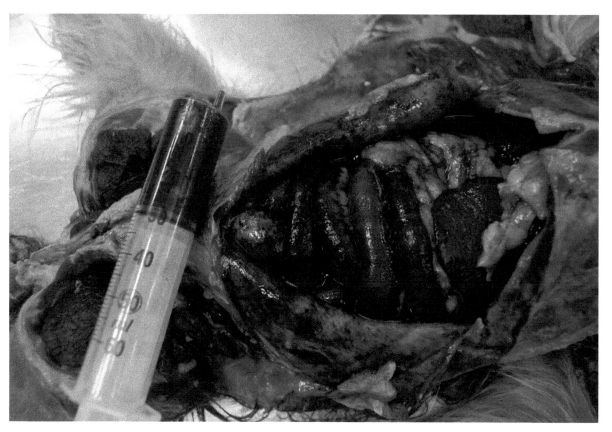

Fig. 1.3 Practice example 2.

4. Keep the body cool (preferably refrigerated) until ready to begin. Do not freeze unless this is completely unavoidable.

## Sampling technique

1. Set out all your tools, water and disinfectant before beginning the necropsy (see the 'Necropsy tools' box). If you need to rinse or flush organs/tissues, always use cold water. You might find it helpful to have a container of hot water handy with detergent for washing your hands periodically, particularly if a sink is not immediately available.
2. Always follow the same necropsy protocol. Approaches vary a little, but most follow a similar process. Our standard protocol is provided at the end, along with references to other approaches.
3. Handle tissues gently (e.g. do not rub mucosal surfaces or overhandle the lungs prior to sampling). As a general rule, when sampling visceral tissues such as liver, kidney or spleen ensure that one dimension is no thicker than a pencil, to allow formalin penetration (this obviously does not apply to organs that are collected whole, particularly the brain).
4. Sample pots should have a wide neck and be large enough to hold the sample plus sufficient neutral buffered formalin (ratio 10:1 of formalin:sample).
5. We take a wide range of tissues routinely from our necropsies (see protocol below). This may not always be practical but, for every necropsy, at the very least sample major visceral organs (liver, lung, heart, kidneys). Sampling of representative samples of the gastrointestinal tract, trachea, muscle, lymph node, spleen, skin, peripheral nerve and endocrine glands is also strongly advised. Look at the brain grossly and retain for histopathology (whole in formalin) if it is abnormal or there have been clinical signs indicative of neurological disease. Sample all grossly abnormal tissue.
6. If you plan to submit samples to an external laboratory for histopathology, it is worth collecting different organs in different smaller pots for clarity. For paired organs, some prosectors will section the left organ longitudinally ('L and L') and the right transversely.
7. Always label pots clearly with animal ID and tissues contained within. Use a screw top container and place in sealable, leak-proof, plastic bags surrounded by absorbent material such as cotton wool. All associated documentation should be in a separate bag. Avoid the use of sticky tape around the lid of the container; it is not very effective and the other measures mentioned are better.
8. Take detailed notes and photographs as necessary.
9. Consider taking fresh samples perhaps for freezing particularly if there is a possibility of toxin exposure (best samples to collect are liver, kidney, stomach content, blood, urine and fat; brain can be helpful). Bear in mind that freezing can affect viability of some organisms so this may affect culture results further down the diagnostic path.

---

Necropsy toolkit

Scissors, preferably blunt-ended

Necropsy knives

Forceps

Clamps/string (for the gastrointestinal tract [GIT])

Scalpel blades and handles

Ruler

Camera

Hacksaw

Syringes and measuring cylinders

Optional: Rongeurs, rib cutters (helpful for larger dogs)

## Report writing

- Your report should include the following information: Necropsy ID # or owner's name; clinic # where applicable; clinician; pathologist/prosector; and date of necropsy.
- Our suggested approach is to write the necropsy report in the past tense and divide it into sections as follows.

  - **First paragraph:** Introductory section outlining signalment (age, breed/predominant breed, species, sex, coat colour), nutritional status (emaciated, thin, lean, good, overweight, obese), postmortem condition (degree of autolysis: excellent, very good, good, adequate, marginal, poor), and weight. Any other identifying features should be noted at this point (e.g. microchip number, tattoo number, ear tag); e.g. 'Presented for necropsy (or postmortem examination) was a 10Y old, neutered male, tricoloured Beagle dog in good nutritional condition and marginal postmortem condition. The body weighed 13.5 kg.' You can use this initial paragraph to include external features, such as skin lacerations, ectoparasites, areas clipped of hair, catheter sites, yellow sclera. Also include the oral cavity, teeth, gingiva, abnormal external lymph nodes, joints and bone marrow findings. This is not meant to be prescriptive – you may want to address these elements in other areas or even at the end – just try to be consistent and you will not forget; a check sheet is recommended.
  - **Second paragraph:** This is a summary of the next body cavity you enter (usually the abdomen, but it may vary with the protocol you use). Note the volume, colour and consistency of any fluid and describe any abnormalities in abdominal organs. Include amount, colour and consistency of gastrointestinal contents, especially the stomach; note if there are formed faeces in the rectum.
  - **Third paragraph:** The third paragraph is a summary of the thoracic cavity. Record the presence or absence of negative pressure in the thoracic cavity, as well as the volume, colour and consistency of any free fluid. In puppies and kittens, comment on size/presence/absence of thymus. Note if portions of lung from all lobes sink or float in formalin/water (proxy indicator of aeration). As with abdominal organs, if the heart is enlarged, record its weight, calculate a percentage body weight and state the normal range.[23]
  - **Fourth paragraph:** The last paragraph would include brain/skull/spinal cord/vertebrae/ if any lesions. Also include anything else not covered above. If you only recorded abnormal findings (which is our approach), it is still a good idea to include a sentence such as: 'The remaining organs examined were grossly normal.'

## Morphological diagnoses

We list the morphological (gross) diagnoses in the same order the lesions appear in the main report to avoid inadvertently missing any diagnoses. We then provide a final gross diagnosis, which is the most important finding. However, some prefer to list the morphological diagnoses in order of importance. It really is not critical which approach you choose but try to be consistent.

### Gross diagnosis

Provide a preliminary diagnosis: i.e. what do you think resulted in this animal dying or being euthanised?

### Comment

Good comments sum up the important lesions and clarify age-related or incidental lesions; they should also summarise the likely pathogenesis or explain why a cause of death has not been identified, e.g. carcass autolysed; anaesthetic death where cause is often difficult to identify. You will ultimately develop your own style, but these are the key features the comment should cover.

> TIP
> - Try to keep body cavities and then organ systems together – discuss gastrointestinal tract, then urogenital tract, then spleen, etc.
> - It is not essential to describe or list normal findings. This is optional. Some pathologists record normal findings, others may simply say 'all other organs within normal limits'. The key is consistency. An equally valid approach is to mention normal findings only when it is pertinent to the case/clinical history; e.g. a dog with a suspected splenic mass on ultrasound but the spleen turns out to be grossly normal.
> - When you suspect organ enlargement, measure and weigh the organ, calculate its percentage of body weight and include in your report, stating the normal range. If this is not available in the literature, measurements may be sufficient.

## Full necropsy protocol

1. Check and record species, breed, sex and colour.
2. Record tattoos/ear tags/microchip.
3. Weigh/estimate weight or body condition.
4. Examine external body, including ears/feet (record abnormalities).
5. Remove and fix both eyes (label L and R in and on pots).
6. Examine hip/stifle/shoulder/elbow joints. Note if synovial fluid is increased in volume or has an altered viscosity/appearance; consider sampling for culture at this stage. Examine skeletal musculature/tendons/ligaments.
7. Collect mandibular lymph node, submandibular salivary gland, skin, testis, mammary tissue, one patella, hind limb skeletal muscle, sciatic nerve and bone marrow. Examine peripheral lymph nodes.
8. Open abdomen, collect and measure peritoneal fluid. Examine viscera in situ (including kidneys and adrenal glands) and note any abnormal vessels, altered organ shape/position.
9. Open diaphragm along costal arch (checking for negative intrathoracic pressure).
10. Open thorax (remove sternum) and pericardial sac, collect and measure any excess pleural/pericardial fluid.
11. **This is a good moment to check the topography of the organs and review the case with a colleague, if appropriate.**
12. Examine and collect both thyroid and adrenal glands (into left and right pots if this is likely to be pertinent to the case).
13. Transect duodenum level with the caudal aspect of the right limb of the pancreas and transect the rectum at the pelvis. Remove the small and large intestine by stripping from the mesentery. Place to one side and keep moist.
14. Dissect out the tongue, examine larynx, cut through hyoid bone and dissect out trachea and oesophagus. Remove with lungs and heart. Examine large pulmonary vessels for thromboemboli.
15. Sample tongue, trachea, oesophagus, all lung lobes and diaphragm (open the oesophagus and trachea along their entire lengths).
16. Open heart (see 'Evaluation of the heart'), rinse out clots, weigh heart. Note size of atria (left should be smaller than right). Measure thickness of both ventricles and, if possible, the interventricular septum (IVS). Fix whole heart if possible or sample both atria, both ventricles, the IVS and valves.
17. Remove stomach with duodenum, liver, gall bladder, spleen* and pancreas. Open the stomach (along lesser curvature) and duodenum (along antimesenteric border). Check patency of bile duct and then separate from liver and spleen. (*Alternatively, remove spleen prior to removing the other organs as this is straightforward to do.)
18. Empty gall bladder, weigh liver. Examine serosal and cut surfaces of liver, spleen and pancreas (serial sections through the parenchyma) and sample pylorus and glandular portion of stomach, duodenum with pancreas, liver, gall bladder and spleen.
19. Open intestinal tract and sample: jejunum (two pieces), ileum, caecum and colon.
20. Check patency of urethra and then remove entire urogenital tract along with remainder of rectum.
21. Longitudinally section kidneys and note corticomedullary ratio; remove capsule and examine surface. Sample kidneys including cortex, medulla and papilla.
22. Examine ureters, urinary bladder and urethra. Sample bladder and any abnormalities.
23. Examine reproductive tract, rectum and anal sacs.
24. Open abdominal aorta to iliac bifurcation and sample, i.e. take a short segment of opened aorta (about 3–4 cm long).
25. Remove brain and pituitary gland, check tympanic bullae (open with rongeurs).
26. Split head and examine nasal cavity.

**DO NOT: Rub mucosal surfaces, over-manipulate tissues, or run tissues under hot water.**

## Evaluation of the heart

### I. Macroscopic evaluation

There is no one way to open the heart but most techniques are variations of a similar approach. Evaluation of the heart is a little like the necropsy – if you open the heart the same way each time, you are more likely to appreciate abnormalities when they crop up. Below is a suggested approach for examination of the heart and preparation of sections for histopathology – it follows the route the blood takes when it enters the heart from the body. Use rounded (not pointed) scissors.

1. Check for pericardial fluid (sample if increased) and open the pericardial sac.
2. Open the heart while still attached to the lungs – this allows you to check for a pulmonary artery thrombus as you can follow the vessel from the heart into the lungs more easily.
3. Snip across the longest axis of the right auricle.
4. The end of this first cut is the start of your next cut into the right ventricle. Aim to cut around the right ventricle as if it is a hip pocket on a pair of trousers.

Start by cutting from the right atrium towards the apex of the heart. You should not actually reach the apex – if you do you have wandered into the left ventricle by mistake. Cut from the apex towards the base of the heart, this time alongside the interventricular septum, and keep going into the pulmonary artery. This allows you to check the pulmonary artery for thromboemboli.

5.  Make a cut similar to that in step 2, but this time across the left auricle.

6.  Slip your scissors into the opened left atrium and slide them into the left ventricle. Cut through the left atrioventricular (AV) valve to open the left ventricle in a line from the left atrium to the apex (i.e. no need to cut around it like the right ventricle).

7.  Slide your scissors under the left AV valve and cut the valve so that the scissors pass on through to the aorta – this is the left ventricular outflow tract and you have completed opening the heart.

8.  If you are happy you have checked for lesions such as a thrombus, thromboembolism or patent ductus arteriosus then trim the great vessels from the heart at the base. Remove blood from the chambers, including clots (remember to keep some of this blood frozen if there is concern regarding exposure to a toxin). Rinse the heart gently with cold water.

9.  Weigh the heart and calculate the percentage of the body weight. For example, a heart weighs 17 g and the cat weighs 4.2 kg. $17/4200 \times 100 = 0.4\%$. Bear in mind that age, sex and nutritional status will influence this to some extent. Normal heart:body weight ratios are provided in the literature for different ages and sexes of dogs and cats.[2,3] They do tend to vary a little but are a good guide. Anecdotally, any heart that weighs more than about 20 g in a standard adult domestic cat has a good chance of being abnormally enlarged and is worth investigating further.

10. For cats, the entire heart can be fixed as a whole organ. For dogs, sections need to be taken and fixed separately.

## II. Trimming the heart for histopathology

1.  Always take samples of both atria, both ventricles and the interventricular septum. Include valves with your sections. It is also worth collecting a transverse section of the left ventricle through the papillary muscle as this is an important conduction area.

2.  Orientation of the atrial sections is not critical, but it can be helpful to take the right atrium with the right ventricle as one long slender piece (no thicker than a pencil). Take the left atrium and left ventricle separately – if you do this every time, you will always know that the piece of atrium on its own is from the left side. A reasonable sample from the left ventricle of a dog might measure approximately 4 cm long and 1 cm wide, the longest dimension running 'with the grain' of the myocardial fibres. Try to include papillary muscle in your samples.

3.  The interventricular septum is a little tricky in smaller hearts due to the curvature of the ventricles – but try to flatten the left ventricle gently and make two cuts (with a knife or scalpel) that are as straight and parallel as possible, to take a section that is about 4–5 cm long and 1 cm wide. These cuts should extend from (and include) the aortic valve and they should be full thickness.

## Brain trimming guidelines

The following outlines a standard approach to taking brain sections appropriate for histopathology. Depending on your place of work, you may only need to remove the brain and fix it prior to submitting it to your chosen veterinary pathology laboratory. In that case, ensure it is well fixed (10% neutral buffered formalin [NBF] is fine) and submit wrapped in absorbent material soaked in 10% formalin (e.g. paper towels or gauze). Place a small amount of NBF in the first plastic bag with the brain and then double bag, with absorbent material around the second bag in case of leakage. Place in a sturdy box for transport. Whether or not you are going to be trimming the brain yourself, ensure the brain has been fully immersed in 10% NBF for at least 5 days – preferably 1 week. If it is still pink on cut section, it is not ready for processing.

### I. Evaluate the external surface of the brain grossly (Fig. 1.4)

You should also do this thoroughly prior to fixing as the formalin will change the colour of the brain. Examine all surfaces, including the ventral aspect, brain stem and optic chiasm. The brain in Fig 1.5 includes leptomeninges but not the dura mater, which usually remains adhered to the calvaria. Note the straight caudal aspect of the cerebellum in this image, which is normal.

### II. Take standard sections of brain (Figs 1.5–1.12)

Serially section at ~5–10 mm intervals as you go, which will allow you to evaluate the parenchyma of the brain. The images below show the minimum number of routine sections that should be selected.

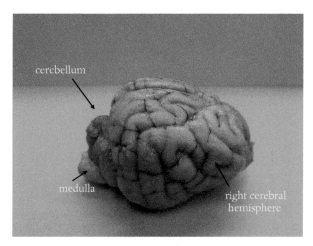

Fig. 1.4

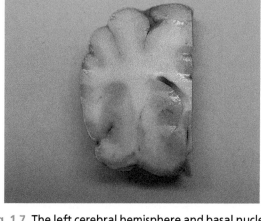

Fig. 1.7 The left cerebral hemisphere and basal nucleus were selected for further processing in this case.

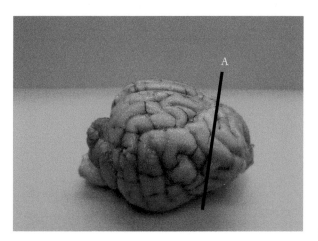

Fig. 1.5 Start at the rostral end of the brain and take this first section at a slight angle to allow for curvature of the hemisphere.

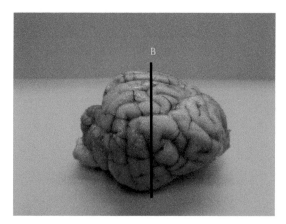

Fig. 1.8

The next routine section is taken approximately through the midpoint of the cerebral hemispheres (Figs 1.8 and 1.9). It should capture the thalamus and hippocampus. Take one-half – the opposite side to that taken at point A is the best approach, otherwise you will only be examining one side of the brain histologically.

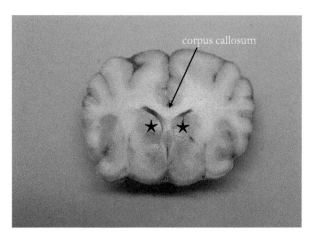

Fig. 1.6 Section taken at point A in Fig. 1.5, at the level of the basal ganglia.

One-half is usually sufficient for further processing assuming there are no grossly apparent lesions. It does not really matter whether you choose left or right side for routine pathological surveillance of the brain (Fig. 1.7). However, as you progress through your sectioning choose alternate sides.

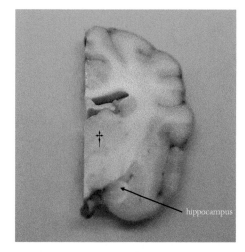

Fig. 1.9 Right cerebral hemisphere with thalamus (†) and hippocampus.

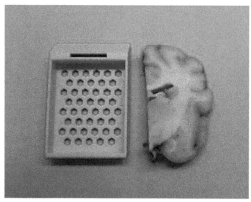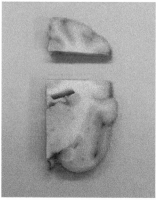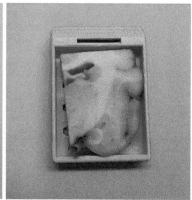

Fig. 1.10. If the section needs to be trimmed to fit the cassette, 'sacrifice' cortex to allow evaluation of hippocampus and thalamus.

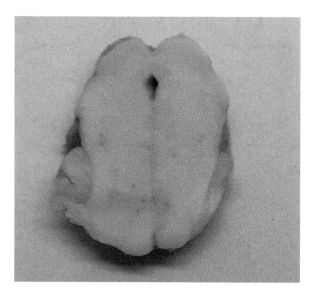

Fig. 1.11 Midbrain. This section is a little asymmetrical, but this is artefactual.

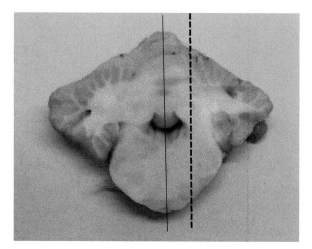

Fig. 1.12 Cerebellum and medulla.

To fit the cassette, you can just take half of the cerebellum and medulla – if possible, trimming at the dashed line in Fig. 1.12 and processing the 'bigger half' to the left side of

the dashed line would be better as it would allow better evaluation of the midline.

Also consider taking a longitudinal section of the cerebellum (i.e. in a rostrocaudal direction), which allows appreciation of any compression of the vermis. While used more commonly in farm animal species, it can be a helpful section to take, particularly if there is concern of cerebellar herniation.

## Approach to necropsy of the neonatal puppy

### Aetiology of canine neonatal death

Canine neonatal death is defined as death of a puppy in the first 6 weeks of life.[4] Approximately two-thirds of deaths occur in the first week of life and about one-half of these are stillbirths.[5] A cause of death is often not identified (more than 50% in some studies) but frequently cited causes include dystocia, low birth weight, congenital defects, trauma, and fading puppy syndrome.[4,6] Infectious disease accounts for a small percentage of deaths. The neonatal puppy is enormously vulnerable for a number of reasons. The following is not an exhaustive list, but it highlights the main causes. The neonate's cardiovascular and renal systems are immature, leaving it prone to collapse, low blood pressure and dehydration.[4] Second, the puppy's liver possesses a finite supply of glycogen that will only sustain it for 24 hours at best if it fails to suckle straightaway.[4] Finally, due to an inability to shiver, the puppy is susceptible to hypothermia; even for normal neonates, this susceptibility may be exacerbated by poor maternal instinct/neglect, lack of colostrum and/or low environmental temperature. Neonates that are already weak may not be able to establish and maintain physical contact with their mother for sufficient periods of time.

### Fading puppy syndrome

This is still not well understood and a single accepted definition has not been established. Some consider it to be a clinical syndrome while others regard it as a diagnosis of exclusion after a full necropsy and in full knowledge of maternal and kennel-based factors.[6,7] Clinically, these puppies are born healthy but weaken over a 2 week period, losing their ability to suckle, becoming weak and recumbent, with paddling, crying and, ultimately, death. Some dams may have multiple affected litters, highlighting the importance of gathering a clinical history that does not focus merely on the current litter or, indeed, only on the puppies.[7,8] Several maternal factors can impact on the success of raising a healthy litter (e.g. the mother's age, behaviour, infections, underlying metabolic or endocrine disease, stress) and environmental factors may also contribute.[4]

## Necropsy approach

Hopefully, the summary above illustrates the need to conduct a full necropsy in any neonatal puppy death investigation, in much the same way as would be pursued in an adult. The necropsy approach used in adults can be easily applied to puppies, ensuring no system is overlooked (see 'Necropsy and tissue sampling: general guidelines'). Modifications in equipment are few – a scalpel is the tool of choice rather than a knife, and smaller scissors and forceps will minimise tissue artefact. Protocol adaptations include assessment and sampling of any submitted placenta, the umbilicus and thymus. Pay close attention to congenital lesions, although bear in mind that not all congenital lesions will cause death. A complete standard adult necropsy protocol should include assessment of joints and bone marrow, and these are also important in the puppy. In addition to sampling of tissues for histopathology, fresh samples should also be collected, suitable for bacterial culture. Appropriate samples are liver, lung, spleen, kidney and placenta. Ideally, ship these on ice within 24 hours. Tissues can be frozen if there is unavoidable delay but bear in mind that this can affect viability of certain organisms, e.g. Campylobacter. Certain infectious causes of abortion in puppies may be associated with neonatal death. They include canine herpesvirus, *Brucella canis*, and the genera *Leptospira*, *Salmonella*, *Campylobacter*, *Streptococcus* and *Neospora*. It is beyond the remit of this book to cover this area in detail, but several more expansive resources are suggested in the references. Lamm and Njaa[8] provide particularly comprehensive and practical guidelines.

## Approach to forensic necropsy cases

A forensic necropsy is required if there may be criminal or civil proceedings following the death of an animal.[9] This is a specialist discipline, which has been expanding over recent years and, in 2020, the European College of Veterinary Pathologists created a Certificate in Forensic Pathology.[10] Before undertaking a forensic case, it is essential that the veterinary surgeon involved has the required qualifications and experience of the species to present the case to a court.[9] A detailed discussion of the approach to a forensic case is beyond the scope of this book and there are journal articles and text books that give more detailed accounts including antemortem investigation, several of which are listed below in the references.[9–12] Some key points to consider are the following.

1. Before undertaking the case, ensure you and your facility are equipped to carry out the full necropsy and to retain all evidence as required by the court.
2. Detailed and accurate records of everything that happens to the submitted animal from the point of receipt to the point of release of the body must all be maintained. This will include dates, times, methods of storage, personnel present at the necropsy and samples retained. Records should be signed and dated to maintain an accurate and traceable chain of evidence.
3. Retain all labels, packaging, digital images from the case and contemporaneous notes until the case is completed.
4. Radiographs prior to commencing the necropsy may be advisable (e.g. to identify acute or chronic fractures; or to localise gunshot pellets or pellet fragments).

## General health and safety considerations

When deciding whether to perform a necropsy, you should consider whether you have sufficient time and resources to complete the task. It is important to ensure the safety of the individual(s) carrying out the procedure and to ensure that no other members of staff or animals are exposed to potentially injurious agents. Take into account the health status of individual staff, e.g. consider the risk of infectious agents or exposure to formalin fumes for potentially immunosuppressed or pregnant individuals.

## Before the necropsy

- Ensure there is adequate space and ventilation to carry out the procedure, with hot and cold running water available.
- Ensure that the necropsy will be performed in an area that is easily cleaned and disinfected.
- Always review the clinical history and consider potential zoonoses/toxins. In some cases, it may not be possible to perform the necropsy safely and consultation with an external laboratory may be advisable. For instance, most diagnostic laboratories will only conduct necropsies on psittacine birds if they have a safety cabinet, which protects from potentially zoonotic disease.

## During the necropsy

Suitable personal protection equipment (PPE) should be worn. The minimum requirement would be protective clothing (including footwear) that can be washed/disinfected (e.g. boiler suits and rubber boots) and disposable gloves. Eye protection and/or facemasks or even respirators may also be advisable e.g. if there is concern of a zoonotic infection, such as leptospira or salmonella. Double gloving or cut proof gloves (if available) are also recommended for any potentially zoonotic cases. All equipment and PPE should be cleaned and disinfected after each case in an appropriate disinfectant.

Gloves should be cleaned of blood/body fluid frequently during the necropsy; perforated or split gloves should be changed and replaced with new gloves after washing hands.

Containers of formalin should be kept covered at all times to protect you and others from fumes, and the containers should be leak proof. Samples for microbiology should also be placed in leak-proof containers.

Consider the risks carefully if asked to undertake a necropsy on a known or suspected mycobacterium case as the possibility of infection with *Mycobacterium bovis* has to be borne in mind. If you unexpectedly find lesions that may be mycobacterium, stop the necropsy immediately. You may still be able to take restricted samples to confirm the suspicion but, depending on findings, relevant animal health authorities may need to be informed. It is possible to conduct molecular typing on fixed tissue if required at a later stage, but mycobacterial culture is strictly controlled.

## After the necropsy

All disposable PPE should be placed in the appropriate clinical waste bin (with special attention to sharps such as blades and needles). The body should be placed in a leak-proof bag and labelled for appropriate disposal (e.g. routine or private cremation). External surfaces of all sample containers should be disinfected at the end of the necropsy and all retained samples should be stored in an appropriate location e.g. chill room, freezer, formalin at room temperature, etc.

## Correlation of cases with Royal College of Veterinary Surgeons (RCVS) Day One Competences

| Competency* | Relevant cases |
|---|---|
| A | MS1, COMPLEX1, COMPLEX3, CNS5 |
| B | HEP9, URIN5, HAEM2 |
| C | COMPLEX1 |
| D | CVS3, CVS10, CVS11, CVS12, CVS13, CVS14, GIT1, GIT3, GIT5, GIT8, GIT10, GIT12, RESP1, RESP4, RESP10, RESP11, HEP2, HEP5, HEP7, HEP8, URIN3, URIN5, URIN8, URIN11, URIN12, MS1, HAEM1, HAEM2, HAEM3, HAEM4, HAEM5, HAEM6, HAEM9, COMPLEX2, REPRO8, CNS1, CNS2, CNS6, END4 |
| E | RESP5, HEP7, HEP9, URIN4, MS1, MS7, COMPLEX2, CNS2, CNS5 |
| F | CVS3, CVS5, CVS9, CVS13, CVS14, GIT3, GIT7, GIT11, RESP1, RESP5, RESP8, RESP9, HEP1, URIN1, URIN6, URIN7, MS1, HAEM3, HAEM6, HAEM8, REPRO1, CNS5, CNS8, END2 |
| G | HEP9, URIN5, HAEM2 |
| H | HEP9, URIN5, HAEM2 |

* Corresponding competences below.

## RCVS Day One Competences relevant to this book[†]

10. Demonstrate self-awareness of personal and professional limits, and know when to seek professional advice, assistance and support [A]
16. Promote health and safety of patients, clients and colleagues in the veterinary setting, including applying the principles of risk management to practice [B]
21. Communicate clearly and collaborate with referral, diagnostic and other professional services [C]
24. Synthesises and prioritises problems to arrive at differential diagnoses [D]
31. Collect, preserve and transport samples, select appropriate diagnostic tests, interpret and understand the limitations of the test results [E]
36. Perform a systematic gross postmortem examination, record observations [F]

40. Recommend and evaluate protocols for biosecurity, and apply principles of biosecurity correctly, including sterilisation of equipment and disinfection of clothing [G]

44. Promote the health and safety of people and the environment [H]

†Numbered directly from RCVS Day One Competences.[13]

## References

1 Law, M., Stromberg, P., Meuten, D. & Cullen, J. (2012) Necropsy or autopsy? It is all about communication! *Veterinary Pathology*, 49, 271–272. https://doi.org/10.1177/0300985811410722

2 McDonough, S.P., & Southard, T. (Eds.) (2016). *Necropsy guide for dogs, cats, and small mammals*. Wiley. http://doi.org.10.1002/9781119317005.

3 Robinson, W. F., & Robinson, N. A. (2016). Cardiovascular system. In M. G. Maxie (Ed.), *Jubb, Kennedy and Palmer's pathology of domestic animals* (6th ed), Vol. 3 (pp. 13). Elsevier. https://doi.org/10.1016/B978-0-7020-5319-1.00012-8

4 Ogbu, K. I., Ochai, S. O., Danladi, M. M. A., Abdullateef, M. H., Agwu, E. O., & Gyengdeng, J. G. (2016). A review of Neonatal mortality in Dogs. *International Journal of Life Sciences*, 4(4), 451–460.

5 Lawler, D. F. (1989). Care and diseases of neonatal puppies and kittens. In Kirk (Ed.), *Current veterinary therapy*, X (pp. 1325–1333). W. B. Saunders Company.

6 Blunden, A. S. (1986). A review of the fading puppy syndrome (also known as fading puppy complex). *Veterinary Annual, 26*, 264–269.

7 Sturgess, K. (1998). Infectious diseases of young puppies and kittens. In G. M. Simpson, G. C. W. England & M. Harvey (Eds.), *Manual of small animal reproduction and neonatology* (pp. 159–166). British Small Animal Veterinary Association.

8 Lamm, C. G., & Njaa, B. L. (2012). Clinical approach to abortion, stillbirth, and neonatal death in dogs and cats. *Veterinary Clinics of North America. Small Animal Practice, 42*(3), 501–513. https://doi.org/10.1016/j.cvsm.2012.01.015

9 Munro, R., & Munro, H. (2011). Forensic veterinary medicine. *In Practice, 33*, 262–270. https://doi.org/10.1136/inp.d3599

10 Munro, R., Ressel, L., Gröne, A., Hetzel, U., Jensen, H. E., Paciello, O., & Kipar, A. (2020). European forensic veterinary pathology Comes of Age. *Journal of Comparative Pathology*, 179, 83–88. https://doi.org/10.1016/j.jcpa.2020.08.003

11 Merck, M. (Ed.) (2013). *Veterinary forensics: Animal cruelty investigations*. John Wiley & Sons.

12 Munro, R., & Munro, H. M. C. (2008). Animal abuse and unlawful killing: Forensic veterinary pathology/Ranald Munro, Helen M. C. Munro. *Print*. Saunders Elsevier.

13 https://www.rcvs.org.uk/news-and-views/publications/rcvs-day-one-competences-feb-2022/

# Cardiovascular system cases

2

# CVS1

## Topics

**Lesion recognition**

**Integration of pathological findings with clinical aspects**

## History

This heart was from a 9Y old, male intact German Shepherd crossbreed dog that collapsed while out for a walk. It was taken to the local veterinary surgeon but was dead on arrival.

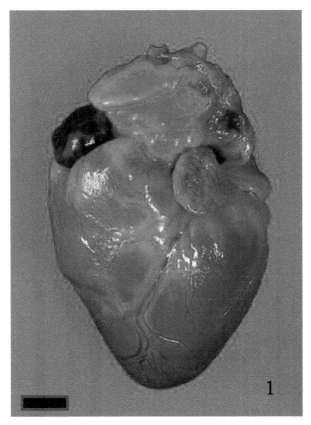 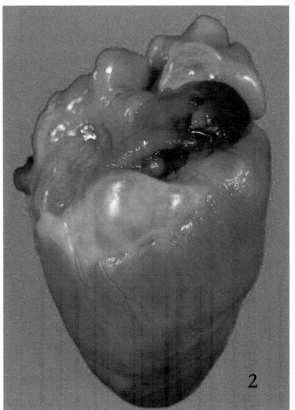

Figs 2.1 and 2.2  Bar = 1 cm. Image credits: Alistair Cox.

## Questions

1. Describe any abnormalities.
2. Provide a diagnosis.
3. What is the **most likely** cause of this dog's death?

# CVS2

## Topics

Lesion recognition

Prioritisation of findings

Integration of pathological findings with clinical aspects

## History

A 6Y old, male intact Rhodesian Ridgeback dog was submitted for necropsy with a 3 day history of lethargy, anorexia and loss of condition. Clinical findings included severe lameness associated with a swollen and painful right elbow, pyrexia, a systolic murmur over the mitral valve and intermittent ventricular tachycardia. The most significant haematological findings consisted of marked peripheral leucocytosis, neutrophilia and thrombocytopaenia (but no evidence of anaemia). The dog died during hospitalisation. Necropsy confirmed suppurative arthritis and synovitis in the right elbow joint. All other joints were grossly normal but there were severe renal infarcts in both kidneys. Fig. 2.3 is an image of the heart from this dog.

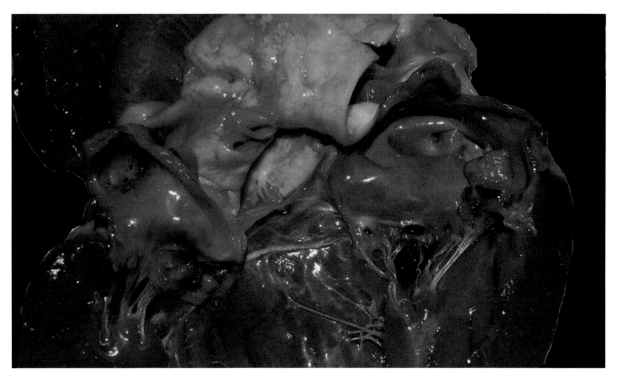

Fig. 2.3

## Questions

1. Describe any abnormalities.
2. Provide a diagnosis.
3. How would you integrate the clinical history with the main pathological findings?

# CVS3

## Topics

Lesion recognition

Pathogenesis

Practical technique

## History

An otherwise healthy, 4Y old, mixed-breed, intact male terrier dog died unexpectedly in transit to the UK (by road). It was submitted for necropsy. The most significant finding (and likely cause of death) is illustrated in Fig. 2.4.

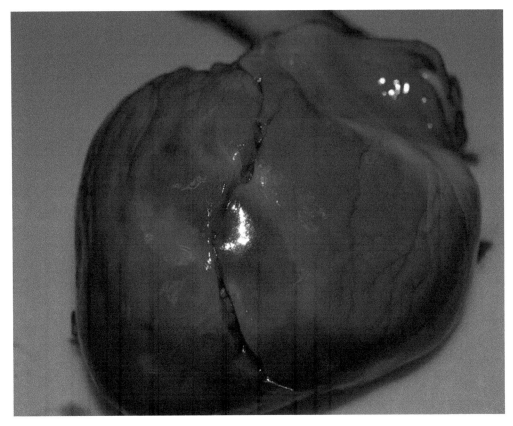

Fig. 2.4

## Questions

1. Describe any abnormalities.
2. Provide a diagnosis.
3. Outline some potential causes of this lesion.

# CVS4

## Topic

Common artefacts and pitfalls

## History

Partially dissected heart from the necropsy of a 6Y old, male Jack Russell Terrier that was euthanised following a road traffic accident.

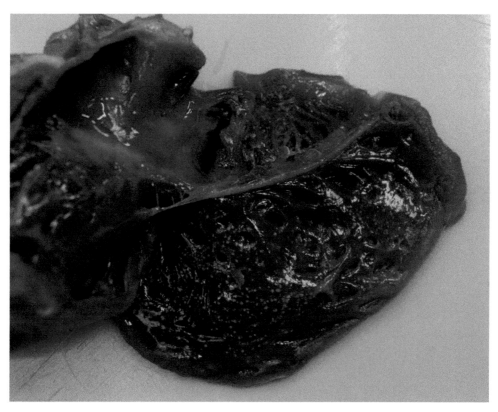

Fig. 2.5

## Questions

1. Describe any abnormalities.
2. Provide a diagnosis.
3. Define the term 'artefact' in the context of pathology.

# CVS5

## Topics

**Lesion recognition**

**Practical technique**

**Pathogenesis**

**Approach to difficult cases**

## History

A fully vaccinated, 10Y old, mixed-breed, male neutered dog was submitted for necropsy following sudden unexpected death. The only reported clinical finding was age-related osteoarthritis in the hips, which was being treated with corticosteroid therapy. The most significant necropsy finding was in the heart (Fig. 2.6). There was a moderate serous effusion in the peritoneal cavity and mild pallor of the renal cortex in both kidneys, but all other organs were grossly normal.

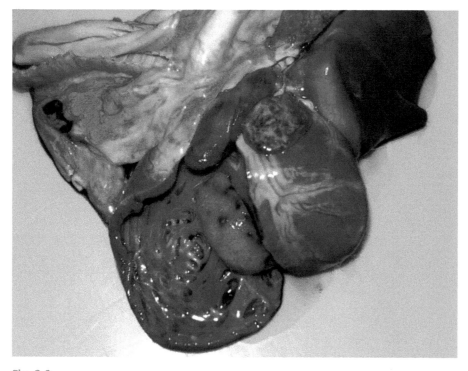

Fig. 2.6

## Questions

1. Describe any abnormalities.
2. Provide a diagnosis.
3. Based on the history provided, outline a potential underlying cause for the lesion in this case.

# CVS6

## Topics

Lesion recognition

Prioritisation of findings

## History

A 10Y old, female spayed Cocker Spaniel presented for necropsy following euthanasia due to a rapidly progressing oral melanoma. Fig. 2.7 depicts another macroscopic abnormality found at necropsy.

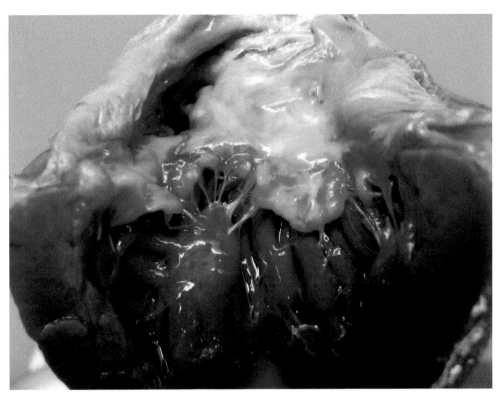

Fig. 2.7

## Questions

1. Describe any abnormalities.
2. Provide a diagnosis.
3. What pathological factors, if present, would help to decide the significance of this lesion?

# CVS7

## Topics

**Lesion recognition**

**Prioritisation of findings**

**Pathogenesis**

## History

The image in Fig. 2.8 illustrates a cardiac finding during the necropsy of a 9Y old, female spayed Boxer.

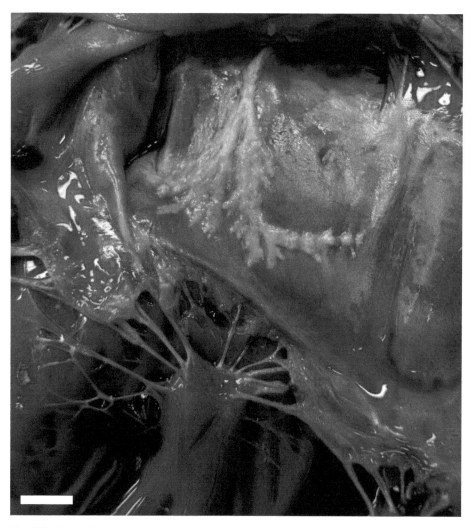

Fig. 2.8 **Bar = 1 cm.**

## Questions

1. Describe any abnormalities.
2. Provide a diagnosis.
3. How would you explain this lesion and where would you look next?

# CVS8

## Topics

Lesion recognition

Common artefacts and pitfalls

## History

Necropsy lesions discovered in an 8Y old, female Labrador with a history of vomiting and lethargy.

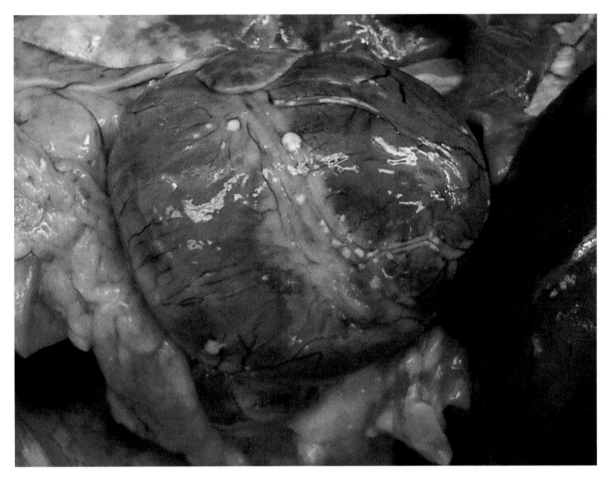

Fig. 2.9

## Questions

1. Describe any abnormalities.
2. Provide a diagnosis.
3. If, for some reason, this was the first lesion you saw at necropsy, where would you make sure to look next?

# CVS9

## Topics

Lesion recognition

Practical technique

## History

A female intact Pug puppy presented at 5 months of age stunted, with breathing difficulties and a continuous heart murmur. For humane reasons it was euthanised. The main necropsy finding is illustrated in Figs 2.10 and 2.11.

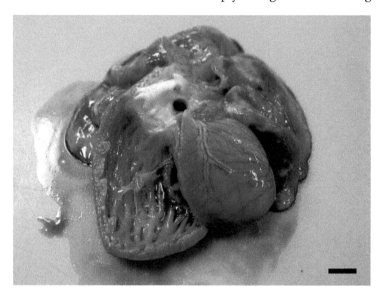

Fig. 2.10  Bar = 1 cm.

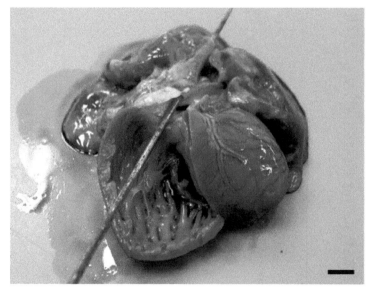

Fig. 2.11

## Questions

1. Describe any abnormalities.
2. Provide a diagnosis.
3. Clue: When should the vessel highlighted by the probe in Fig. 2.11 close in the dog?

# CVS10

## Topics

Lesion recognition

Generation of pathological differential diagnoses lists

## History

Fig. 2.12 depicts one of many gross abnormalities in an 8Y old, male neutered Siamese cat that had metastatic lymphoma and had to be euthanised on humane grounds.

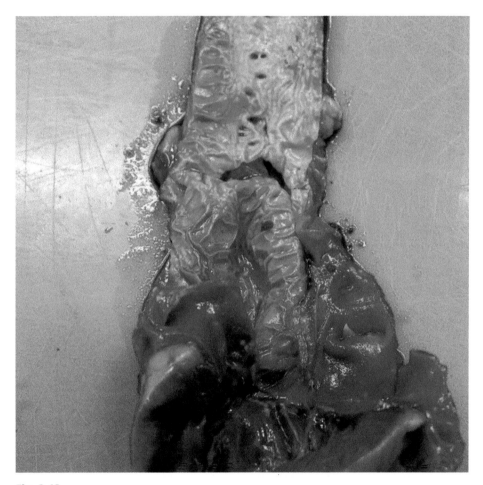

Fig. 2.12

## Questions

1. Describe any abnormalities.
2. Provide a diagnosis.
3. How would you link this lesion to the history in this case? Outline some other potential causes of this lesion.

# CVS11

## Topics

- Lesion recognition
- Prioritisation of findings
- Integration of pathological findings with clinical aspects
- Pathogenesis

## History

A 6Y old, female domestic longhaired cat was euthanised following a period of sudden onset paresis progressing to recumbency that was unresponsive to therapy. The image in Fig. 2.13 illustrates the most significant gross necropsy findings.

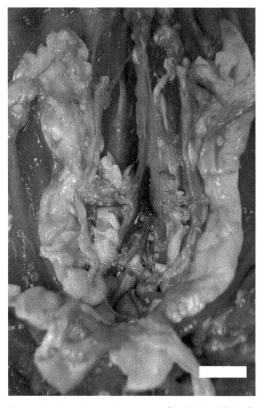

Fig. 2.13  Bar = 1 cm. Image credit: Dr David Walker.

## Questions

1. Describe any abnormalities in Fig. 2.13.
2. Provide a diagnosis.
3. This lesion is usually secondary, i.e. an indicator of disease elsewhere. Provide some differentials for possible underlying causes (aim to provide at least **FOUR**).

# CVS12

## Topics

Lesion recognition

Generation of pathological differential diagnoses lists

Pathogenesis

## History

A 9Y old, male intact Boston Terrier was submitted for necropsy following a period of lethargy, inappetance, ascites and identification of a mediastinal mass on imaging.

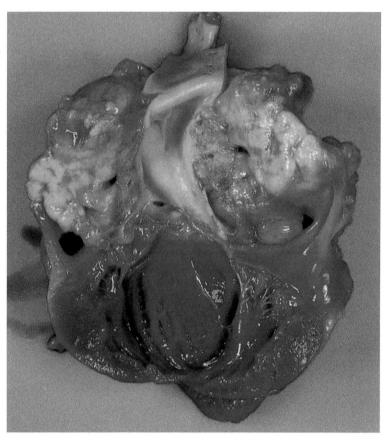

Fig. 2.14

## Questions

1. Describe any abnormalities.
2. Provide a diagnosis.
3. As this lesion compromises cardiovascular function, list some other changes you might expect to find at necropsy.

# CVS13

## Topics

Practical technique

Lesion recognition

Generation of pathological differential diagnoses lists

## History

A 3Y old, female neutered Maine Coon cat was found dead a few days after it had returned home from a stay at a cattery while its owners were away. The main gross finding was in the heart, illustrated in Fig. 2.15 (formalin-fixed). The heart weighed 37 g (normal is approximately 18–20 g although a comparative ratio is more helpful, especially in large breeds i.e. comparison of heart weight to body weight).

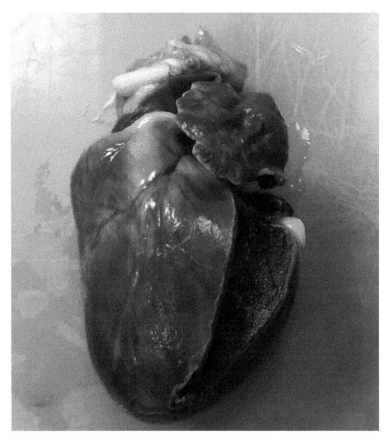

Fig. 2.15

## Questions

1. Describe any abnormalities.
2. Provide a diagnosis.
3. Outline some possible causes of cardiomegaly in the cat.

# CVS14

## Topics

Practical technique

Lesion recognition

Generation of pathological differential diagnoses lists

## History and signalment

A 3Y old, male crossbreed dog was submitted for necropsy after a spell of lethargy with episodes of collapse and decreased appetite. It died on the way to the veterinary practice for a consultation. Fig. 2.16 shows the macroscopic appearance of the heart.

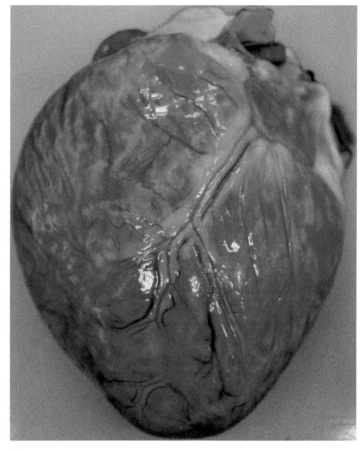

Fig. 2.16

## Questions

1. Describe any abnormalities.
2. Provide a diagnosis.
3. Suggest some possible causes of the pathological changes.

# CVS1 answers

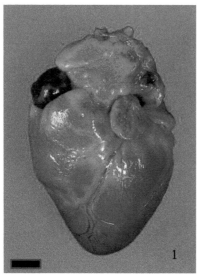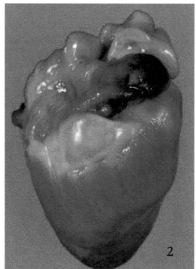

Figs. 2.1 and 2.2 **Bar = 1 cm.**

## 1. Describe any abnormalities

The right atrial appendage is distorted and thickened by a focal, dark red, ill-defined, irregular mass that measures approximately 3 × 2 cm.

## 2. Provide a diagnosis

This is a right atrial/auricular haemangiosarcoma, a highly aggressive malignancy classically considered to be of endothelial cell origin, although recent research suggests that it may in fact derive from a pluripotent bone marrow progenitor cell.[1–3] Haemangiosarcoma accounts for almost 70% of primary cardiac tumours in the dog but cardiac tumours are rare in general (overall incidence of 0.19%).[4] Susceptible breeds include Golden Retrievers and German Shepherd dogs.[5] This example is fairly obvious but it is worth bearing in mind that this tumour can sometimes be quite subtle, manifesting as much smaller areas of red, rough epicardium over the right auricle. Other commonly affected sites in the dog are the liver, spleen and skin/subcutis.

## 3. What is the **most likely** cause of this dog's death?

In this case the dog collapsed suddenly and, given the location of the lesion, the haemangiosarcoma likely ruptured, leading to haemorrhage into the pericardial sac. Cardiac tamponade would probably cause death before hypovolaemia. Visceral haemangiosarcomas may present as haemoabdomen rather than sudden death. Other potential mechanisms of death with this malignancy include pneumonia, disseminated intravascular coagulopathy and arrhythmias.[6]

## References

1 Cohen, S. M., Storer, R. D., Criswell, K. A., Doerrer, N. G., Dellarco, V. L., Pegg, D. G., Wojcinski, Z. W., Malarkey, D. E., Jacobs, A. C., Klaunig, J. E., Swenberg, J. A., & Cook, J. C. (2009). Hemangiosarcoma in rodents: Mode-of-action evaluation and human relevance. *Toxicological Sciences, 111*(1), 4–18. https://doi.org/10.1093/toxsci/kfp131

2 Gorden, B. H., Kim, J. H., Sarver, A. L., Frantz, A. M., Breen, M., Lindblad-Toh, K., O'Brien, T. D., Sharkey, L. C., Modiano, J. F., & Dickerson, E. B. (2014). Identification of three molecular and functional subtypes in canine hemangiosarcoma through gene expression profiling and progenitor cell characterization. *American Journal of Pathology, 184*(4), 985–995. https://doi.org/10.1016/j.ajpath.2013.12.025

3 Kim, J. H., Graef, A. J., Dickerson, E. B., & Modiano, J. F. (2015). Pathobiology of hemangiosarcoma in dogs: Research advances and future perspectives. *Veterinary Sciences, 2*(4), 388–405. https://doi.org/10.3390/vetsci2040388

4 Ware, W. A., & Hopper, D. L. (1999). Cardiac tumors in dogs: 1982–1995. *Journal of Veterinary Internal Medicine, 13*(2), 95–103. https://doi.org/10.1111/j.1939-1676.1999.tb01136.x

5 Yamamoto, S., Hoshi, K., Hirakawa, A., Chimura, S., Kobayashi, M., & Machida, N. (2013). Epidemiological, clinical and pathological features of primary cardiac hemangiosarcoma in dogs: A review of 51 cases. *Journal of Veterinary Medical Science, 75*(11), 1433–1441. https://doi.org/10.1292/jvms.13-0064

6 Aronsohn, M. (1985). Cardiac hemangiosarcoma in the dog: A review of 38 cases. *Journal of the American Veterinary Medical Association, 187*(9), 922–926.

# CVS2 answers

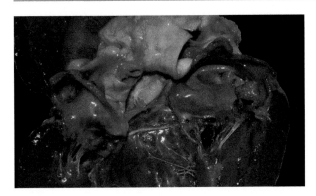

Fig. 2.3

## 1.   Describe any abnormalities

There is moderate multifocal nodular thickening of the mitral valve leaflets (see Fig. 2.3a). The nodules are irregular, pale pink or red and verrucous, ranging up to 1.5 cm diameter. There is also a transverse band of white, fibrous tissue, approximately 2 mm wide and 3 cm long, on the endocardial surface of the subaortic outflow tract, approximately 1 cm below the aortic valve.

> Note that the aortic valve is grossly normal; the leaflets are not completely opened in the image.

## 2.   Provide a diagnosis

a.   Moderate multifocal subacute vegetative valvular endocarditis – mitral valve.

b.   Subaortic stenosis.

## 3.   How would you integrate the clinical history with the main pathological findings?

The vegetative endocarditis is the most significant finding in terms of the clinical presentation. It is uncommon in dogs, especially compared to other domesticated species, but has been linked to a number of bacterial organisms, including *Streptococcus* spp., *Staphylococcus aureus* and *Escherichia coli*.[1] It explains the mitral valve murmur and,

since one of the risks is thromboembolism, also accounts for the renal infarcts. Thrombocytopaenia is most likely due to excessive consumption since this dog was probably affected by sepsis-induced disseminated intravascular coagulopathy (DIC). Leucocytosis, neutrophilia and pyrexia reflect bacterial infection and likely also tissue necrosis. Inflammation of joints is often associated with sepsis and/ or vegetative endocarditis since it is a consequence of bacteraemia and seeding of bacteria to one or more joints. Of course, the infected joint may be the initial source of infection. Subaortic stenosis is an inherited congenital condition in the dog but there is a belief in practice that it may make the adjacent aortic valve vulnerable to bacterial infection spreading via the haematogenous route from, for example, areas of periodontal disease, cystitis, etc.[1,2]

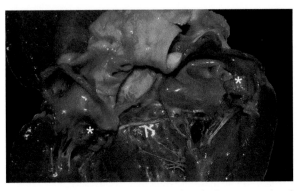

Fig. 2.3a **Canine heart. Vegetative lesions on mitral valve (*) and subaortic stenosis (arrowhead).**

## References

1   MacDonald, K. (2010). Infective endocarditis in dogs: Diagnosis and therapy. *Veterinary Clinics of North America. Small Animal Practice*, 40(4), 665–684. https://doi.org/10.1016/j. cvsm.2010.03.010

2   Robinson, W. F., & Robinson, N. A. (2016). Cardiovascular system. In M. G. Maxie (Ed.), *Jubb, Kennedy and Palmer's pathology of domestic animals* (6th ed), Vol. 3 (pp. 20–21). Elsevier. https://doi.org/10.1016/B978-0-7020-5319-1.00012-8

# CVS3 answers

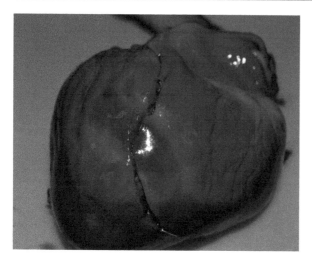

Fig. 2.4

have seen other similar cases of myocardial infarction in the canine heart in recent years, with no underlying vascular disease identified. Nonetheless, myocardial necrosis has the potential to lead to fatal arrhythmias and cardiogenic shock.

> TIP
>
> Fig. 2.4a depicts a myocardial infarct in the left ventricle of a different dog (also an unexpected death). This case highlights the importance of serially sectioning ('bread-loafing') the myocardium of the heart, especially in sudden death cases, though it is good practice to do this in every case. It is entirely possible for there to be a myocardial infarct that is only appreciable on cut section.

### 1. Describe any abnormalities

There is a well-demarcated, focal, rectangular, rust-red/brown lesion on the epicardial surface of the right ventricle. This is circumferentially surrounded by a pale tan rim measuring up to ~5 mm thick. While not obvious from the image, this lesion extended into the myocardium.

### 2. Provide a diagnosis

Severe, focal, acute, myocardial infarct (the pale tan rim suggests an acute inflammatory infiltrate in response to the necrosis, which can begin to occur within a few hours).

### 3. Outline some potential causes of this lesion

Although common in humans, myocardial infarcts are rare in the dog. In humans, they are often associated with primary vascular disease, particularly atherosclerosis, although other contributing factors often play a role.[1] Atherosclerosis is recognised in the dog but is usually associated with specific underlying conditions such as hypothyroidism and diabetes mellitus.[2] A small percentage of canine myocardial infarct cases in the veterinary literature have been linked to valvular disease.[3] The thyroid glands in this dog were grossly normal and the blood vessels were histologically within normal limits, with no evidence of vasculitis, atherosclerosis, arteriosclerosis or thrombosis. Heart valves were also grossly normal. The triggering reason for the infarct in this dog is therefore uncertain but we

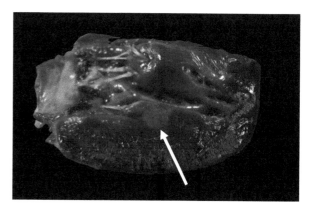

Fig. 2.4a  **Myocardial infarct, canine heart (arrow).**

### References

1  Malakar, A. K., Choudhury, D., Halder, B., Paul, P., Uddin, A., & Chakraborty, S. (2019). A review on coronary artery disease, its risk factors, and therapeutics. *Journal of Cellular Physiology*, 234(10), 16812–16823. https://doi.org/10.1002/jcp.28350

2  Hess, R. S., Kass, P. H., & Van Winkle, T. J. (2003). Association between diabetes mellitus, hypothyroidism or hyperadrenocorticism, and atherosclerosis in dogs. *Journal of Veterinary Internal Medicine*, 17(4), 489–494. https://doi.org/10.1111/j.1939-1676.2003.tb02469.x

3  Driehuys, S., Van Winkle, T. J., Sammarco, C. D., & Drobatz, K. J. (1998). Myocardial infarction in dogs and cats: 37 cases (1985–1994). *Journal of the American Veterinary Medical Association*, 213(10), 1444–1448.

# CVS4 answers

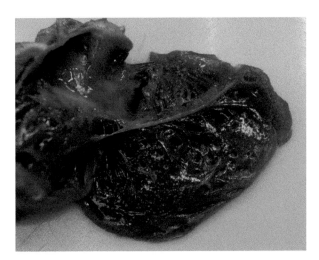

Fig. 2.5

## 1. Describe any abnormalities

The only abnormality comprises multiple, pinpoint, white foci scattered over the endocardial surface of the right atrium and ventricle. On very close inspection, the white foci have a fine 'starburst' or stellate shape. They are not actual lesions, however. Rather, they are barbiturate crystals arising from the method of euthanasia and they may be scattered over any internal surface of the body, though generally the thoracic cavity. They can feel slightly gritty. Fig. 2.5a and b below depict similar crystals in two different cases.

## 2. Provide a diagnosis

Diagnosis: Euthanasia artefact.

There is no true pathological diagnosis as the heart is effectively normal. The barbiturate crystals are a common artefact of euthanasia but it is important not to mistake them for a true lesion.

## 3. Define the term 'artefact' in the context of pathology

An artefact in pathology can be macroscopic (grossly appreciable) or microscopic. It is something structurally appreciable that is artificial and extraneous, generally added after death, during decomposition or processing of tissues (see case GIT8). Examples may include discolouration of tissues due to autolysis or freeze/thaw artefact; increased friability of tissues; and gas distension of organs due to autolysis etc. Artefacts can also occur histologically,

whether introduced around the time of sampling (e.g. crushing the tissue with forceps; poor fixation) or at time of processing in the laboratory (e.g. microtome 'chatter' artefact; folding of tissues).[1]

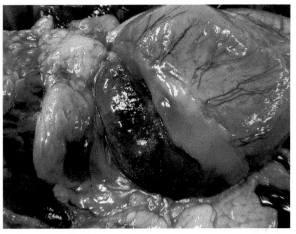

Fig. 2.5a Barbiturate crystals over the epicardial surface of the right auricle.

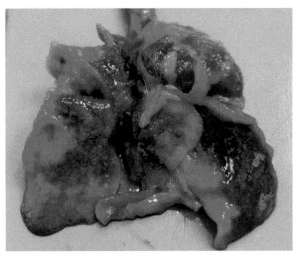

Fig. 2.5b Barbiturate crystals on the pleural surface of a puppy's lungs and pericardium.

## Reference

1 McInnes, E. (2005). Artefacts in histopathology. *Comparative Clinical Pathology*, *13*(3), 100–108. https://doi.org/10.1007/s00580-004-0532-4

# CVS5 answers

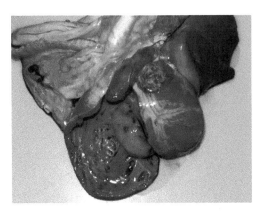

Fig. 2.6

## 1.   Describe any abnormalities

The image illustrates a red, slightly roughened, cylindrical structure within the pulmonary artery. It measures approximately 1.5 cm in diameter and at least 4 cm long. A second similar, wedge-shaped structure lies below it within the right ventricle.

> In general, postmortem clots are dark red to purple, smooth, shiny and easily detached.

## 2.   Provide a diagnosis

Right ventricular and pulmonary artery thromboembolism (PTE).

## 3.   Based on the history provided, outline: (a) a potential underlying cause for the lesion in this case; and (b) how this would have led to death

a.   PTE is generally due to an imbalance in the levels of pro- and anticoagulants, such that coagulation is favoured. A number of predisposing factors can do this but, in this case, one factor that stands out is the corticosteroid treatment for the osteoarthritis. Cortisol predisposes the recipient to a pro-coagulant state so it is likely that iatrogenic hypercortisolism is the cause of the PTE in this case. The role of cortisol in the hypercoagulable state is not entirely clear but a number of associated abnormalities are evident which result in functional hypercoagulability (increased fibrinogen, Factor VIII, Factor IX, and von Willebrand factor [vWF]). There is also reduced fibrinolysis, which tilts the balance further towards coagulation. Other potential underlying causes of PTE (in general, not necessarily in this particular case) include sepsis, immune-mediated haemolytic anaemia, neoplasia,

cardiovascular disease and protein-losing nephropathy. The moderate peritoneal effusion was likely due to hypertension related to heart failure. The renal pallor may have been a postmortem change or a reflection of hypoxia leading to acute tubular necrosis, but histological assessment would help to clarify and rule out other differentials.

b.   Blockage of the pulmonary artery and its branches leads to hypoxia. Blood fails to reach the lungs for oxygenation and, the closer the thrombus is to the heart, the more severe the hypoxia and the quicker the death. Hypoxia would be accompanied by systemic hypotension and cardiovascular collapse.

A similar lesion is shown in Fig. 2.6a, this time from a 4Y old, female neutered Persian cat that died during a routine dental procedure. Thrombosis could be linked to sepsis arising from severe dental/periodontal disease, since sepsis is a potential and common cause of disseminated intravascular coagulopathy. However, in cats, cardiomyopathy is a frequent underlying cause.

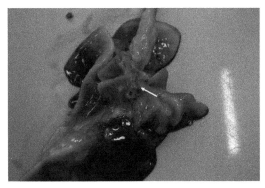

Fig. 2.6a Lung from a cat with pulmonary artery thromboembolism (arrow).

> **TIP**
>
> Leave the heart attached to the lungs to allow you to open the pulmonary artery as it exits the heart and enters the lungs. This is the easiest way to identify pulmonary artery thromboembolism and is an important part of the necropsy, particularly in a case of sudden or unexpected death.

## Reference

1  Caswell, J. L., & Williams, K. J. (2016). Respiratory system. In M. G. Maxie (Ed.), *Jubb, Kennedy and Palmer's pathology of domestic animals* (6th ed), Vol. 2. Elsevier. https://doi.org/10.1016/B978-0-7020-5318-4.00011-5

# CVS6 answers

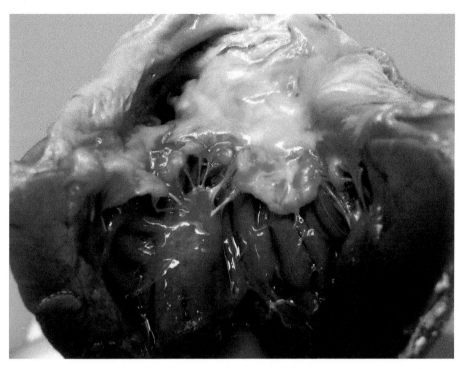

Fig. 2.7

## 1. Describe any abnormalities

There is multifocal nodular thickening of the mitral valve leaflets. The nodules are smooth, shiny and pale pink. They coalesce to form a plaque-like thickening on the anterior (aortic) leaflet (*). The left ventricular wall is thicker than normal, as is the papillary muscle. These latter features are more difficult to appreciate from the image, but the papillary muscle does appear 'fatter' or broader than normal.

## 2. Provide a diagnosis

a. Mitral valve endocardiosis.

b. Marked myocardial hypertrophy (cardiomegaly).

> Endocardiosis is graded into four groups (1 to 4).[1,2] This example is severe and correlates with at least grade 3.

## 3. What pathological factors, if present, would help to decide the significance of this lesion?

Endocardiosis is the most common cardiovascular disease in dogs and it tends to increase with age. Certain breeds are predisposed. The Cavalier King Charles Spaniel is probably best known but other toy and small breeds are vulnerable, as is the Cocker Spaniel used in this example. Any valve may be affected but mitral valves are involved in well over

50% of cases in some studies, sometimes in combination with other valves. At necropsy, valve thickening is more likely to be clinically significant if there is extension of the thickening to the chordae tendinae, subsequent rupture of the chordae tendinae, or jet lesions (areas of subendocardial fibrosis above the valve due to turbulence; see CVS7).[2] Higher grade lesions are also more likely to be clinically significant and other significant changes within the heart may include any of the following: atrial dilation, hypertrophy and dilation of the ventricles, diffuse endocardial fibrosis (white discolouration of the endocardium), and/or atrial mural thrombi etc. Advanced cases may progress to congestive heart failure, for which classic necropsy findings include cavity effusions (e.g. ascites), pulmonary oedema and chronic passive congestion of the liver. Right-sided heart failure may lead to cavity effusions and peripheral oedema, while left-sided heart failure leads to pulmonary oedema[2].

## References

1  Pomerance, A., & Whitney, J. C. (1970). Heart valve changes common to man and dog: A comparative study. *Cardiovascular Research, 4*(1), 61–66. https://doi.org/10.1093/cvr/4.1.61

2  Borgarelli, M., & Buchanan, J. W. (2012). Historical review, epidemiology and natural history of degenerative mitral valve disease. *Journal of Veterinary Cardiology, 14*(1), 93–101. https://doi.org/10.1016/j.jvc.2012.01.011

# CVS7 answers

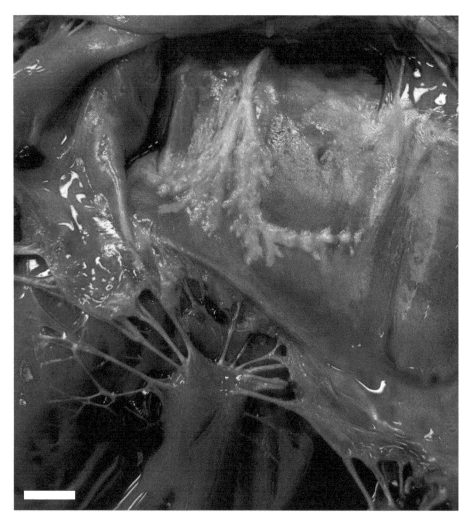

Fig. 2.8 Bar = 1 cm.

## 1.   Describe any abnormalities

On the endocardial surface of the left atrium there is a slightly raised, pale fawn to white, irregularly linear, arborising lesion that spans an area measuring ~3 × 4 cm.

> We know this is the left side of the heart because of the size of the papillary muscle.

## 2.   Provide a diagnosis

Moderate, focally extensive, endocardial fibrosis ('jet' lesion) – left atrium.

## 3.   How would you explain this lesion and where would you look next?

Jet lesions usually form due to valvular incompetence, leading to back flow (or regurgitation) from the ventricle to the atrium. The regular spouting pressure of the regurgitated blood onto the atrial endocardium causes endothelial damage with deposition of fibrin and platelets. Eventually this will repair by fibrosis, the reparative collagen following the path of the endothelial damage. So, it would be important to examine the valves next, in this case the mitral valve. There was no evidence of endocarditis or endocardiosis in this dog but valvular incompetence was diagnosed, since some chordae tendinae were shorter than normal (not obvious from the image). The dog also had chronic passive congestion in its liver, supportive of heart failure.

# CVS8 answers

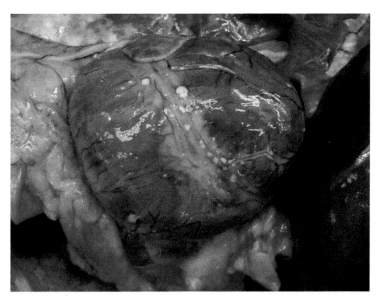

Fig. 2.9

## 1. Describe any abnormalities

There are multifocal, coalescing, white, flat, chalky plaques on the epicardial surface of the heart. They range in diameter up to approximately 5 mm.

## 2. Provide a diagnosis

Moderate multifocal acute epicardial fat necrosis with saponification and mineralisation.

## 3. If, for some reason, this was the first lesion you saw at necropsy, where would you make sure to look next?

The pancreas. The white, chalky lesions over the epicardial fat are foci of fat necrosis and the most likely cause of this in a dog is acute pancreatic necrosis (also known as necrotising pancreatitis). Involvement of pericardial fat is more unusual but do not forget to look at the pancreas when you see this type of lesion. In some animals, the fat necrosis may present as dermal nodules due to panniculitis. Fig. 2.9a depicts a more typical presentation. See also case HEP10.

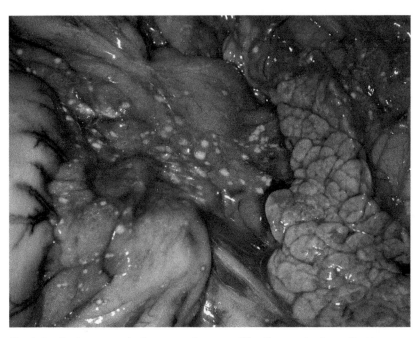

Fig. 2.9a Peripancreatic fat necrosis, saponification and mineralisation.

# CVS9 answers

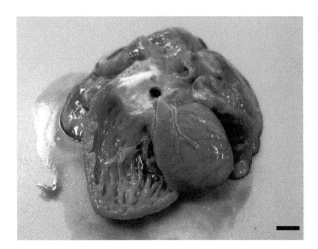

Fig. 2.10  Bar = 1 cm.

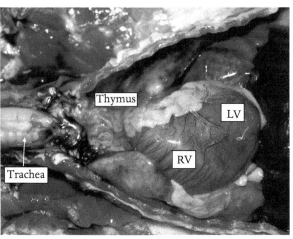

Fig. 2.10a  Thoracic cavity, 5-month-old Pug. The thymus tells us this is a young dog.

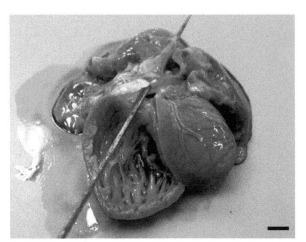

Fig. 2.11

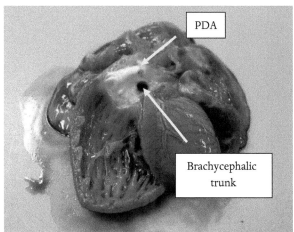

Fig. 2.11a  Heart, 5-month-old Pug.

## 1.  Describe any abnormalities

There is a patent vascular connection between the pulmonary artery and, just behind it, the aorta. It measures approximately 1–2 mm diameter. The right ventricle is mildly dilated (more obvious in Fig. 2.10a).

## 2.  Provide a diagnosis

Patent ductus arteriosus (see Fig 2.11a).

## 3.  Clue: When should the vessel highlighted by the probe in Fig 2.11 close in the dog?

The ductus arteriosus closes within hours of birth, at least in terms of its function, as the tunica media contracts and closes the lumen.[1] The consequences of a PDA include (usually) left-to-right shunting of blood with subsequent left atrial dilation, left ventricular eccentric hypertrophy (i.e. thickened wall with concurrent ventricular dilation), right ventricular concentric hypertrophy (i.e. thickened wall only with no chamber dilation), cardiomegaly, arrhythmias and congestive heart failure.[1]

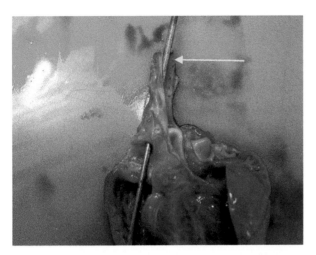

**Fig. 2.11c.** Heart, 5-month-old Pug. The probe lies within the PDA linking the pulmonary artery to the aorta. The arrow denotes the aorta. The small regular holes in this vessel are arterial branches leaving the aorta – they are not present in the pulmonary artery so help to identify the aorta. The entrance to the brachycephalic trunk appears enlarged – the reason is unclear but we speculated this may be breed related.

**Reference**

1  Robinson, W. F., & Robinson, N. A. (2016). Cardiovascular system. In M. G. Maxie (Ed.), *Jubb, Kennedy and Palmer's pathology of domestic animals* (6th ed), Vol. 3 *(pp. 17–18)*. Elsevier. https://doi.org/10.1016/B978-0-7020-5319-1.00012-8

---

**TIP**

As mentioned in other cases, it is always advisable to leave the heart and lungs attached prior to opening the heart so that you can check major vessels, particularly the pulmonary artery, for thromboemboli.

A further advantage is that this will allow evaluation of the relationships of the vessels and easier identification of any abnormalities. So, it is always best to leave long lengths of the aorta and pulmonary artery intact until you can check for lesions such as PDA. You can remove these when you want to weigh the heart.

Also check that the oesophagus or trachea are not entrapped prior to removing the pluck* from the thorax – i.e. check for a vascular ring anomaly too.

*pluck = heart and lungs

# CVS10 answers

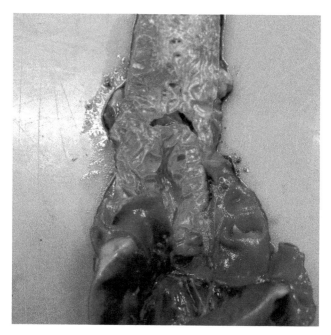

Fig. 2.12

## 1.   Describe any abnormalities

The ascending aorta is diffusely thickened and very irregular with formation of folds that confer a 'wrinkled' appearance. The left ventricle of the heart is also moderately thickened.

## 2.   Provide a diagnosis

a.  Severe diffuse aortic mineralisation.

b.  Moderate left ventricular hypertrophy.

## 3.   How would you link this lesion to the history in this case? Outline some other potential causes of this lesion

This is a manifestation of soft tissue mineralisation. Mineralisation of the soft tissues may be dystrophic or metastatic. Dystrophic mineralisation follows necrosis and may occur in areas of inflammation, degeneration or ischaemia. Metastatic mineralisation arises as a result of hypercalcaemia (and also hyperphosphataemia). Lymphoma is a potential cause of hypercalcaemia, but other causes are outlined below:

a.  hyperparathyroidism (parathyroid neoplasia or hyperplasia)

b.  renal disease (mineralisation is a feature of uraemia, particularly in the lungs and the intercostal muscles)

c.  vitamin D toxicosis (more common in ruminants and horses that may ingest excess vitamin D but accidental poisoning can occur in cats exposed to rodenticides containing vitamin $D_3$)

d.  destructive bone disease

e.  paraneoplastic hypercalcaemia (as mentioned above, this can occur with lymphoma; it is perhaps less common in the cat compared to the dog but worth considering during necropsy).

Note: In the dog, Addison's disease can be linked to hypercalcaemia.

TIP

The aorta is recognisable in Fig. 2.12 due to the regular holes in its wall which are off-shoots of various arteries to supply thoracic organs and tissues. This helps to distinguish from the pulmonary artery if you are an anatomy novice (refer to CVS9 too).

This is a far from common lesion in the cat, certainly to this extent, but it is a good opportunity to review general causes of soft tissue mineralisation. Mineral deposition can occur anywhere, not just on the inner surface of the aorta. It may also be recognisable as white chalky deposits.

# CVS11 answers

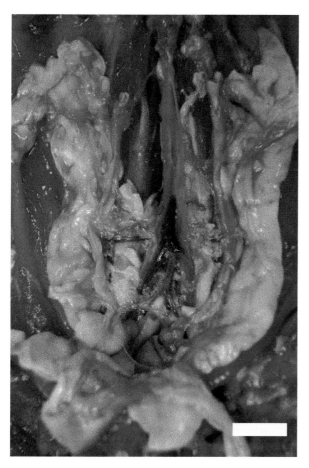

Fig. 2.13 **Bar = 1 cm.**

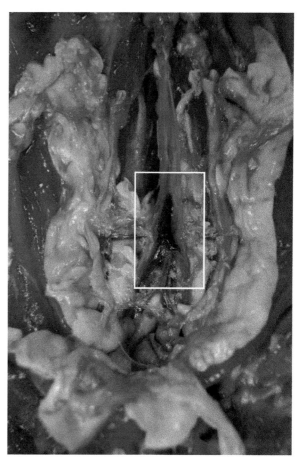

Fig. 2.13a **Caudal abdomen, 6Y old cat.**

### 1.  Describe any abnormalities in Fig. 2.13
Completely occluding the abdominal aorta, near its trifurcation, there is a dark red, segmental, branching structure that measures approximately 2 cm long and 3–4 mm wide (see Fig. 2.13a).

### 2.  Provide a diagnosis
Focal segmental aortic (iliac) thromboembolus ('saddle' thrombus).

### 3.  This is usually a secondary lesion, i.e. an indicator of disease elsewhere. Provide some differentials for possible underlying causes (aim to provide at least **FOUR**)

a.  Cardiac disease (particular cardiomyopathy but also thyrotoxic cardiomegaly) – this is the most common cause in the cat.

b.  Disseminated intravascular coagulopathy – which in turn can have lots of potential causes but the most common is sepsis.

c.  Underlying neoplasia.

d.  Vasculitis.

e.  Protein-losing glomerulopathy.

# CVS12 answers

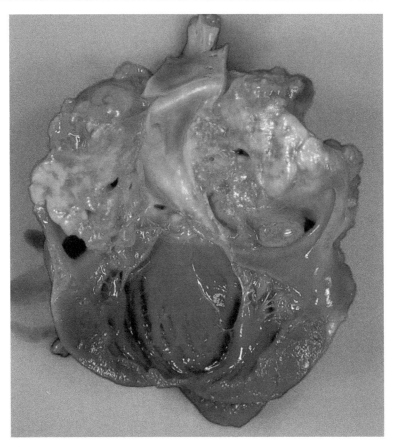

Fig. 2.14

## 1.  Describe any abnormalities

The image is of the heart and aorta as it exits the left ventricle. There is an ill-defined, off-white to pale pink, solid mass surrounding the base of the aorta and obscuring the atria.

## 2.  Provide a diagnosis

The location of the lesion is consistent with a heart base tumour and, in brachycephalic breeds (including the Boston Terrier, Boxer, etc.), an aortic body tumour would be most likely in this location (synonym chemodectoma). Adenomas are generally more common in dogs than carcinomas but these tumours act as space-occupying lesions causing local compression of the surrounding vessels and atria. Carotid body tumours are the other tumour of chemoreceptor organs in the dog but would typically present in the cranioventral region of the neck. Another differential for a mass in this location is an ectopic thyroid carcinoma but these account for <10% of the tumours arising at this site. Lymphoma is also possible, though can usually be distinguished by a softer consistency – it often also bulges on cut section.

## 3.  As this lesion compromises cardiovascular function, list some other changes you might expect to find at necropsy

Hydrothorax, hydropericardium, oedema of subcutaneous tissues of the head and forelimbs and/or passive congestion of the liver. Hydrothorax and hydropericardium are cavity manifestations of oedema and would most likely be due to increased hydrostatic pressure as the lesion compresses surrounding vessels.

# CVS13 answers

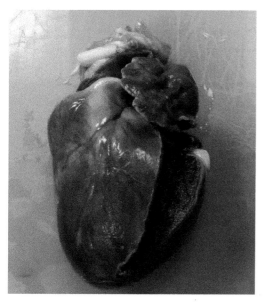

Fig. 2.15

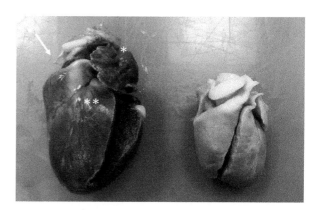

Fig. 2.15a The heart on the left is our case heart; the heart on the right is from a normal cat that died due to a non-cardiac reason (both formalin-fixed): *left auricle; **left ventricle; arrow = right ventricle.

## 1.  Describe any abnormalities

This type of case is trickier to assess from a two-dimensional image, but this heart is enlarged. In Fig. 2.15a the asterisk denotes the left auricle, which is enlarged. While it cannot be seen from the picture, the left auricle was larger than the right auricle, which is an abnormality (the left auricle should be smaller). The right ventricle looks somewhat rounded at the base of the heart (arrow) but this is more subjective and it may be a little displaced or compressed by the left ventricular thickening.

## 2.  Provide a diagnosis

Cardiomegaly. Cardiomyopathy is acceptable as an answer but is really a differential diagnosis of a potential disease that could lead to cardiomegaly. Cardiomegaly is the basic lesion, i.e. enlargement of the heart.

## 3.  Outline some possible causes of cardiomegaly in the cat

This may be the result of hypertrophic cardiomyopathy which implies primary disease of the cardiac muscle, commonly reported in some breeds (including Maine Coons).[1,2] Cardiomegaly could also be caused by hyperthyroidism (thyrotoxic cardiomegaly) or may be secondary to a congenital heart condition, such as mitral valve dysplasia.[3]

Comparing with a normal feline heart helps to appreciate the lesion more convincingly (both cats were a similar bodyweight). The heart on the right is paler, likely because it has been fixed for longer and is less congested than the heart on the left. It is rotated a little compared to the left heart so we can see more of the right ventricle and right atrium.

### TIP: Gross evaluation of the heart

1.  Check for pericardial fluid (sample and measure the fluid if increased) then open the pericardial sac.
2.  Open the heart while still attached to the lungs.
3.  Open as per 'Evaluation of the heart' (Chapter 1). Gently remove blood, including clots, and wash the heart gently with cold water.
4.  Inspect the endocardium, valves, myocardium, epicardium and pericardium for gross lesions.
5.  Weigh the heart and compare to the body weight.
6.  Since the feline heart is small the entire heart can be fixed for histopathology, with sections taken after 2 or 3 days' fixation.

## References

1  Kittleson, M. D., Meurs, K. M., Munro, M. J., Kittleson, J. A., Liu, S. K., Pion, P. D., & Towbin, J. A. (1999). Familial hypertrophic cardiomyopathy in Maine Coon Cats: An animal model of human disease. *Circulation, 99*(24), 3172–3180. https://doi.org/10.1161/01.cir.99.24.3172

2  Kittleson, M. D., & Côté, E. (2021) The Feline Cardiomyopathies: 2. Hypertrophic cardiomyopathy. *Journal of Feline Medicine and Surgery, 23*(11), 1028–1051. https://doi.org/10.1177/1098612X211020162

3  Kittleson, M. D., & Côté (2021) The Feline Cardiomyopathies: 3. Cardiomyopathies other than HCM. *Journal of Feline Medicine and Surgery, 23*(11), 1053–1067. https://doi.org/10.1177/1098612X211030218

# CVS14 answers

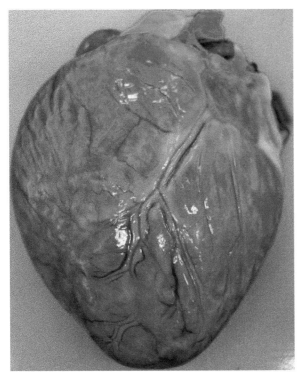

Fig. 2.16

## 1.  Describe any abnormalities

The epicardial surface is mottled due to multifocal to coalescing, pale tan to off-white areas that are sometimes slightly depressed (difficult to see the depressed nature of some of the lesions). If this was your case, you would need to incise into the myocardium to see if the changes extended into the underlying tissue (they did).

## 2.  Provide a diagnosis

Severe, multifocal to coalescing, chronic myocarditis.

Note: The mottling is consistent with myocardial disease but it is not clear if this is due to inflammation, necrosis, mineralisation or a combination of all three. Multifocal depressed areas of myocardium are suggestive of areas of myofibre necrosis and loss with repair by fibrosis (scarring). Scarring indicates chronicity to the changes, despite the short duration of the clinical signs. Necrotic myocardium may also be darker than surrounding viable areas (e.g. as in myocardial infarcts). Fatty infiltration of the myocardium tends to be more homogenously white and may have a greasy texture. Severe mineralisation would be expected to have a gritty texture.

## 3.  Suggest some possible causes of the pathological changes

There are many potential causes of myocarditis in dogs. They include bacteria, viruses, fungi, protozoa, toxins, trauma etc. However, myocarditis may also be part of a generalised myopathy, such as in animals with muscular dystrophy or polymyositis. In this case, the dog had a generalised polymyositis of unknown aetiology identified at the time of necropsy.

TIP

Always open the pericardium and carefully evaluate the epicardial surface of the heart. It can be easy to miss lesions if this is not fully examined and remember that sometimes the macroscopic changes are subtle (unlike this case) and histopathology is worthwhile in any animal with a clinical history of arrhythmia/dysrhythmia or sudden death.

# Gastrointestinal tract cases

3

# GIT1

## Topics

- Lesion recognition
- Generation of pathological differential diagnoses lists
- Integration of pathological findings with clinical aspects
- Pathogenesis

## History

A 9Y old, female neutered Boxer dog died unexpectedly, although there was a vague history of chronic diarrhoea and some weight loss. The dog's last visit to the referring veterinary surgeon was for routine reasons, 6 months previously. The owner requested a necropsy as they were concerned about an underlying infection risk for their other dogs. The pathologist found a gastric dilatation and volvulus and confirmed this as the cause of death. However, they also found some intestinal abnormalities (Fig. 3.1).

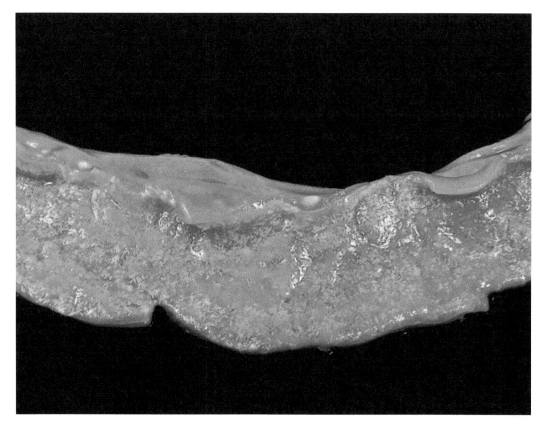

Fig. 3.1

## Questions

1. Describe any abnormalities.
2. Provide a diagnosis.
3. Name **TWO** commonly associated biochemical abnormalities.

# GIT2

## Topics

Lesion recognition

Pathogenesis

## History

A 12Y old, male neutered Cocker Spaniel presented as an out-of-hours emergency referral with acute collapse, a painful abdomen, lethargy and pyrexia. The referring veterinary surgeon also suspected an intra-abdominal mass. The dog had vomited white, frothy liquid several times the previous day. There was a history of dietary indiscretion, enteritis, severe dental disease and arthritis managed with meloxicam. Radiographs and ultrasound confirmed an abdominal mass just caudal to the liver. Although the dog received some supportive treatment, the prognosis was poor and the owner elected for euthanasia and requested a necropsy. The most significant necropsy finding is shown in Fig. 3.2. Fig. 3.3 is a Giemsa-stained smear prepared from ~50 ml of turbid, malodorous, dirty pink peritoneal fluid.

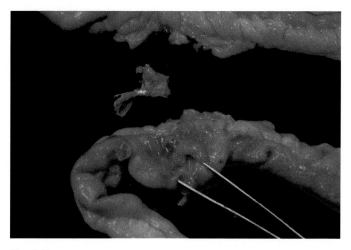

Fig. 3.2

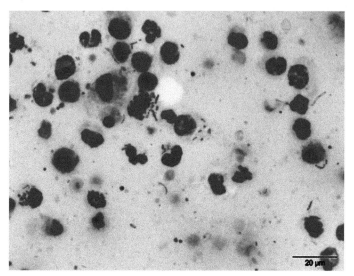

Fig. 3.3

## Questions

1. Describe any abnormalities.
2. Provide a diagnosis.
3. Outline the likely cause of death?

# GIT3

## Topics

Practical technique

Common artefacts and pitfalls

Generation of pathological differential diagnoses lists

## History

A 10Y old, male neutered Doberman was found dead one morning at home, following a short spell of inappetance and lethargy. At necropsy, the most significant lesion was in the abdominal cavity (see Fig. 3.4).

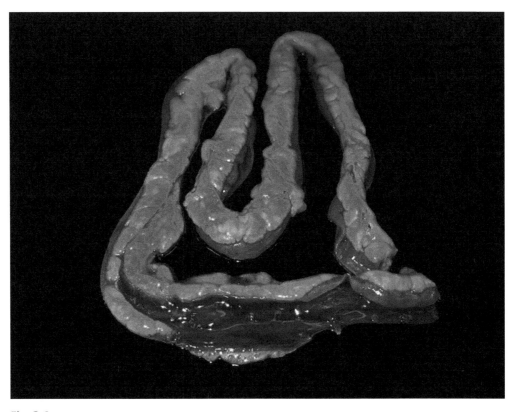

Fig. 3.4

## Questions

1. Describe any abnormalities.
2. Provide a diagnosis.
3. List **FOUR** potential causes.

# GIT4

## Topic

**Lesion recognition**

## History

Following a prolonged period of anorexia, lethargy and weight loss, an 18-month-old, male, domestic shorthair cat was euthanised due to failure to respond to treatment. Pertinent necropsy findings are illustrated in Fig. 3.5.

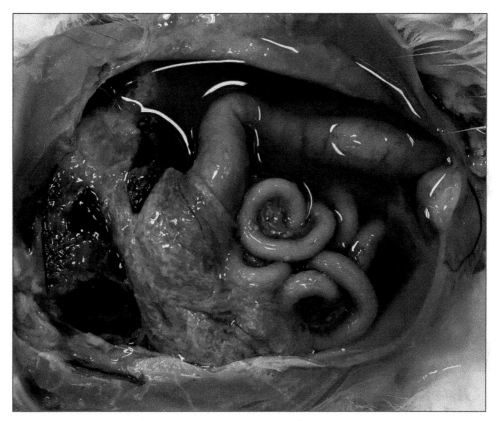

Fig. 3.5 Image credit: Dr Alex Malbon.

## Questions

1. Describe any abnormalities.
2. Provide a diagnosis.
3. Name the disease and the aetiological agent.

# GIT5

## Topics

Lesion recognition

Generation of pathological differential diagnoses lists

Pathogenesis

## History

A 2Y old, male neutered Beagle died following a period of symptomatic treatment for severe, acute vomiting and blood-tinged diarrhoea. Vaccination and worming history were not up to date. The main gross finding is illustrated in Fig. 3.6.

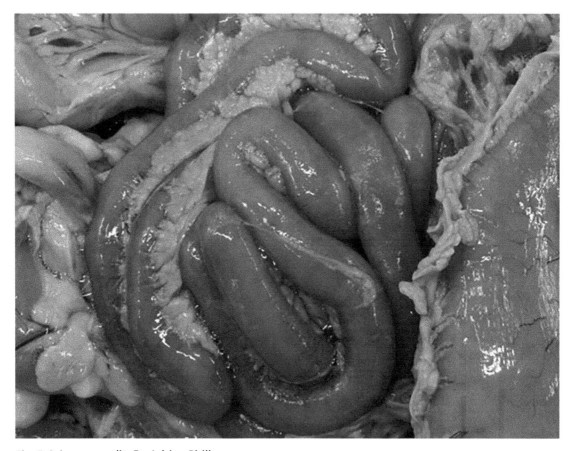

Fig. 3.6 Image credit: Dr Adrian Philbey.

## Questions

1. Describe any abnormalities.
2. Provide a diagnosis.
3. Provide some differential diagnoses for **acute** vomiting and diarrhoea in the adult dog.

# GIT6

## Topics

**Lesion recognition**

**Pathogenesis**

## History

A neonatal, male Rottweiler puppy died after a 36 hour period of gradual fading. The pup never suckled well and failed to pass any meconium or faeces.

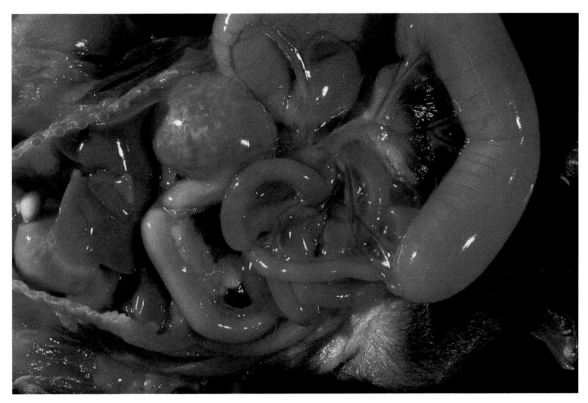

Fig. 3.7

## Questions

1. Describe any abnormalities.
2. Provide a diagnosis.
3. Define atresia (big clue!) and how it differs from stenosis; provide some possible causes of death in this case.

# GIT7

## Topics

Lesion recognition

Pathogenesis

Common artefacts and pitfalls

## History

An adult, female intact Labrador crossbreed dog was submitted for necropsy having been found dead by an animal welfare charity. Neighbours had previously reported that the dog had been tied up in a garden with no food or water. Fig. 3.8 and 3.9 illustrate the main necropsy findings. One additional finding, surprisingly, was that the stomach was full of food.

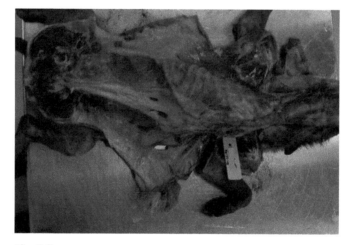

Fig. 3.8

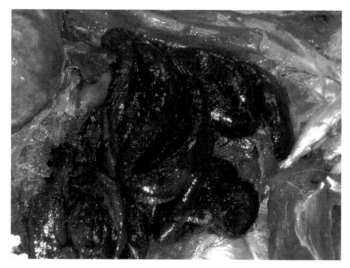

Fig. 3.9

## Questions

1. Describe any abnormalities.
2. Provide a diagnosis.
3. What is the most likely pathogenesis of the lesion in Fig. 3.9?

# GIT8

## Topics

Lesion recognition

Generation of pathological differential diagnoses lists

Pathogenesis

## History

Fig. 3.10 is an image of the opened stomach from the necropsy of an 11Y old, male neutered German Shepherd Dog with a history of abdominal pain, melena and anaemia.

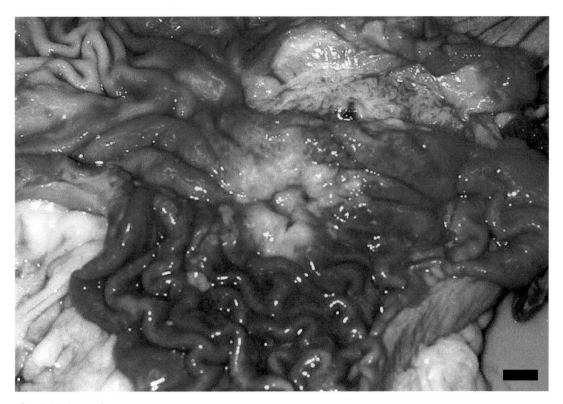

Fig. 3.10  Bar = 1 cm.

## Questions

1. Describe any abnormalities.
2. Provide a diagnosis.
3. List **FOUR** possible causes of this lesion in the dog.

# GIT9

## Topics

**Lesion recognition**

**Integration of pathological findings with clinical aspects**

**Pathogenesis**

## History

A 2Y old, male neutered Bichon Frise was submitted for necropsy after presenting in an obtunded state. The dog died shortly after admission despite supportive therapy. The main necropsy findings are illustrated in Figs 3.11–3.13 below.

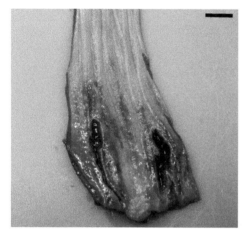

Fig. 3.11 Bar = 1 cm.

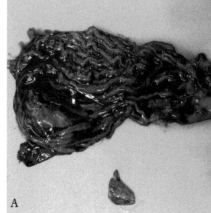
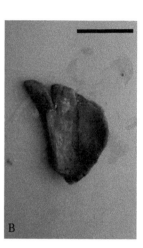

Fig. 3.12 A–B Bar = 1 cm.

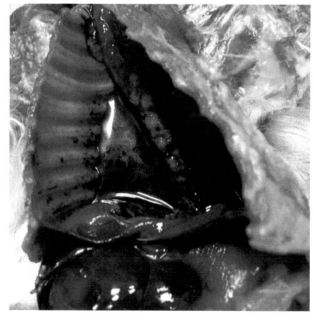

Fig. 3.13

## Questions

1. Describe any abnormalities.
2. Provide a diagnosis/es.
3. Provide a summary to explain the cause of death and pathogenesis of the findings in this dog.

# GIT10

## Topics

Lesion recognition

Common artefacts and pitfalls

Prioritisation of findings

Generation of pathological differential diagnoses lists

Integration of pathological findings with clinical aspects

## History

A 10Y old, male neutered Border Collie presented for necropsy with a history of weight loss, intermittent vomiting, persistently raised liver enzymes, general malaise and inappetence. The dog was non-pyrexic and had responded somewhat to symptomatic treatment, including broad-spectrum antimicrobial therapy, prednisolone and nutritional support. Eventually, however, the clinical response waned, and the owners made the decision to euthanise. There was some concern regarding toxin exposure, hence the request for necropsy. Figs 3.14–3.17 illustrate the most pertinent findings at necropsy (Fig. 3.17 is the stomach).

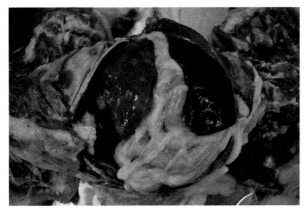

Fig. 3.14

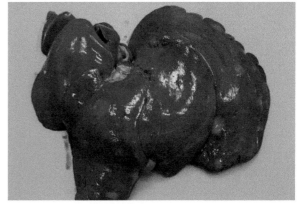

Fig. 3.15

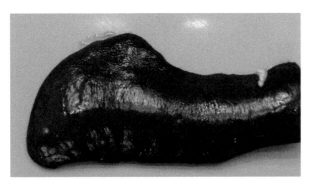

Fig. 3.16

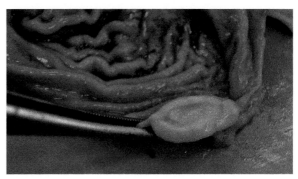

Fig. 3.17

## Questions

1. Describe any abnormalities.
2. Provide a diagnosis/es.
3. a) Given the clinical history, explain the colour and size of the liver.
   b) What is the clinical significance of the splenic changes?
   c) Provide some **non-neoplastic** differentials for the liver nodules.

# GIT11

## Topics

Lesion recognition

Integration of pathological findings with clinical aspects

Pathogenesis

## History

An 8Y old, male neutered Keeshond was found dead in the kitchen one morning by its owners. It was fully vaccinated with no premonitory clinical signs. It was given free access to the enclosed garden and was usually on the lead when out on walks. The main gross finding is illustrated in Fig. 3.18.

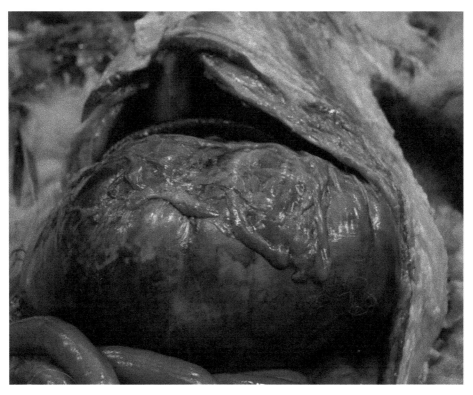

Fig. 3.18

## Questions

1. Describe any abnormalities.
2. Provide a diagnosis.
3. a) Briefly describe what has happened to this stomach, i.e. outline the pathogenesis.
   b) Provide some possible causes.
   c) How might this lead to sudden death, as it did in this case?

# GIT12

## Topics

Lesion recognition

Generation of pathological differential diagnoses lists

## History

A stray cat was found dull, dehydrated and emaciated. It was euthanised on welfare grounds and frozen prior to being submitted for necropsy. The main necropsy findings are shown in Figs 3.24 and 3.25.

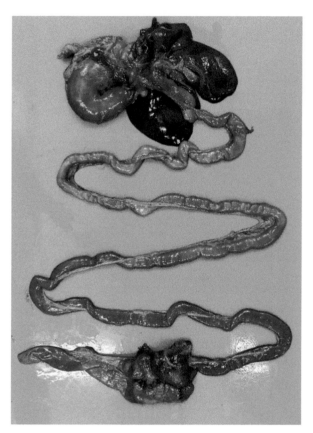

Fig. 3.19

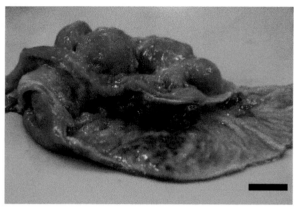

Fig. 3.20  Bar = 1 cm.

## Questions

1. Describe any abnormalities in the images.
2. Provide a diagnosis.
3. In addition to the focal lesion at the ileocaecocolic junction, this cat also had multifocal, white, bulging nodules within the renal parenchyma but no other lesions were macroscopically appreciable. What is the most likely final diagnosis?

# GIT1 answers

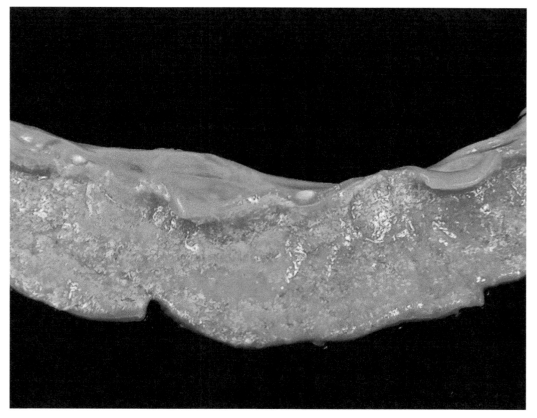

Fig. 3.1

### 1.  Describe any abnormalities

There are myriad slender, short, pale yellow to white, filiform projections over the small intestinal mucosal surface.
There are also at least two smooth, slightly raised, pale
yellow, oval nodules in the wall or submucosa of the small
intestine, measuring up to approximately 4 × 3 mm.

### 2.  Provide a diagnosis

Intestinal lymphangiectasia and granulomatous
lymphangitis.

The filiform projections in Fig. 3.1 correspond to dilated
central villous lacteals; they are white due to stagnation of
chyle. Intestinal lymphangiectasia (dilated lymphatic vessels) can be due to congenital malformation of lymphatic
vessels but many cases are acquired due to obstruction.
In this case, the yellow nodules correspond to lipogranu-
lomas but they are not a consistent finding. It is not clear
whether these granulomas cause obstruction and subsequent rupture or whether they occur secondary to rupture
and release of chyle. Breed predispositions have been rec-

ognised (Soft Coated Wheaten Terrier, Yorkshire Terrier).
In the absence of lymphangiectasia, differentials for the
yellow nodules include metastatic neoplasia, foreign body
granulomas, infectious granulomas (e.g. aberrant parasitic
larval migration; always at least consider *Mycobacterium*
spp.). In cats, feline infectious peritonitis would be a reasonable differential. They are not, however, consistent with
pancreatitis or peripancreatic fat necrosis – in such cases,
lesions are generally flat, white and chalky or opaque and
centred on fat, due to fat saponification.

### 3.  Name TWO commonly associated biochemical abnormalities

Hypoalbuminaemia, hypocalcaemia, lymphopaenia and
hypocholesterolaemia – all due to loss of these nutri-
ents and cells through chyle and protein leakage, as well
as malabsorption. Malabsorption of vitamin D may also
play a role in low calcium levels. As a result of the hypoalbuminaemia, particularly in severe cases, there may be
concomitant oedema and ascites.

# GIT2 answers

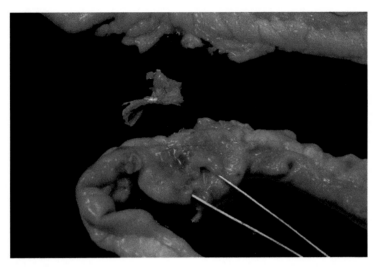

Fig. 3.2

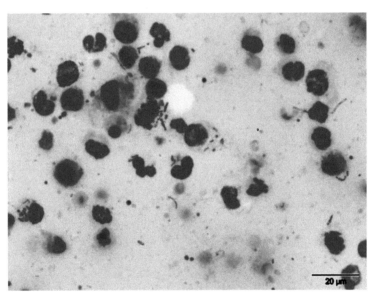

Fig. 3.3

## 1.   Describe any abnormalities

Fig. 3.2: The small intestine (jejunum) is perforated, characterised by a ~2 cm diameter, full-thickness hole in the jejunal wall. The affected area is thinner than normal and almost translucent. The adjacent foreign body originated from the small intestinal lumen and comprises the tip of a paint brush (including the metal band).

Fig. 3.3: The smear consists mainly of degenerate neutrophils (crisp nuclear lobation no longer apparent) and macrophages, with many extracellular and smaller numbers of intracellular bacterial bacilli and cocci.

## 2.   Provide a diagnosis

Intestinal foreign body with focal perforation and septic peritonitis.

## 3.   Outline the likely cause of death?

Septic shock (a form of maldistributive shock) is the likely cause of death. In septic shock, bacteria and their products directly 'switch on' the complement system, neutrophils, the coagulation pathway (via Factor XII) and endothelial cells, stimulating production and release of large amounts of inflammatory mediators (e.g. cytokines, vasoactive amines, kinins) and triggering thrombosis, increased vascular permeability and vasodilation. Working in concert, the inflammatory mediators and exaggerated host response lead to cardiovascular collapse (i.e. reduced blood pressure; haemodynamic abnormalities; reduced tissue perfusion and hypoxia; disseminated intravascular coagulopathy [DIC]; multiple organ failure; then death).

# GIT3 answers

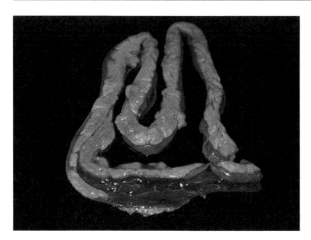

Fig. 3.4

## 1. Describe any abnormalities

The small intestinal mucosa is diffusely dark red and there is scant content other than a small amount of viscous red fluid.

## 2. Provide a diagnosis

Severe, diffuse, mucosal haemorrhage and congestion – small intestine. (Severe haemorrhagic enteritis/enteropathy is an acceptable answer.)

## 3. List **FOUR** potential causes

In addition to haemorrhage and congestion, there may also be inflammation and necrosis in this intestine. The most likely causes are infectious disease or vascular compromise.

### Infectious causes

While more likely in farm animals, *Salmonella* spp., and *Clostridium perfringens* should still be considered. *Escherichia coli* has the potential to cause gastrointestinal disease in the dog but often in conjunction with other infectious agents and not usually associated with sudden unexpected death. Peracute haemorrhagic gastroenteritis (also known as acute haemorrhagic diarrhoea syndrome) is believed to be caused by *C. perfringens* although this is not proven. This essentially idiopathic condition is more common in young (<2Y old) toy and miniature dog breeds. Canine parvovirus type 2 is an important condition to exclude, particularly as the postmortem presentation can vary. Classically, foul smelling, haemorrhagic intestinal content is described, sometimes containing necrotic debris (sloughed mucosa). Since there is often villous atrophy, loss of the normal velvety texture of the mucosa is also a helpful clue. However,

lesions may be subtle, hence the need for histopathology, where crypt necrosis is confirmatory. Protozoa and parasites are more likely to cause more chronic clinical signs, such as diarrhoea and weight loss (any may even result in obstruction in heavy infestations), rather than sudden death with no premonitory signs.

### Vascular compromise

Mesenteric torsion (volvulus) usually occurs at the root of the mesentery and is generally clearly apparent on initial investigation of intestinal orientation. It would result in diffuse acute haemorrhage and necrosis of the entire jejunum. Less extensive, but still well-demarcated, areas of haemorrhage and necrosis may arise if there is volvulus of shorter segments. An important consideration is 'shock gut' which may be higher on the differential list if there is no evidence of primary intestinal infection, volvulus or obstruction. The intestinal tract is one of the major shock organs in the dog. Shock gut is the result of reduced perfusion of vessels supplying the intestinal tract i.e. ischaemia, due to reflex vasoconstriction in response to conditions such as hypovolaemia, heart failure and haemorrhage. You should look for an underlying cause of shock in such cases.

---

TIP

- Use blunt-ended scissors to open the entire gastrointestinal tract (GIT) from oesophagus to rectum – we cut along the ante-mesenteric border but this is not critical.
- Document the character of the content, including whether or not there are formed faeces in the colon and rectum.
- DO NOT RUB the mucosa – you will create artefact and compromise histopathology.
- Take multiple samples from different levels and fix, even if the GIT appears normal. Agents such as parvovirus may affect the GIT in an intermittent pattern so taking multiple levels increases the likelihood of finding histological lesions.
- Prior to fixing, flush excess content away with cold water – agitate gently in water while holding one end with forceps.
- Do not forget potential zoonoses and protect yourself and others.
- Collect a fresh enclosed loop of intestine for bacterial culture to exclude differentials such as *Salmonella*, *Clostridium perfringens* and *E. coli*.

# GIT4 answers

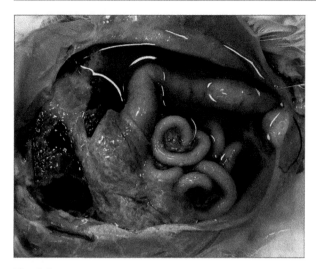

Fig. 3.5

## 1.  Describe any abnormalities

The peritoneal cavity contains a large amount of transparent amber fluid. The parietal peritoneum and the visible surface of the liver are almost completely covered with a membrane of pale yellow/fawn material (fibrin). The omentum is largely devoid of fat reserves but multifocally covered by irregular, coalescing, ill-defined plaques of yellow material that range in diameter up to approximately 0.5 cm. There are several raised, white to pale yellow, smooth, well-defined, nodular plaques on the intestinal serosa.

## 2.  Provide a diagnosis

a.  Severe, diffuse, fibrinous peritonitis with ascites.

b.  Moderate, multifocal, pyogranulomatous intestinal serositis (peritonitis).

## 3.  Name the disease and the aetiological agent

The gross lesions in this case are classic for feline infectious peritonitis (FIP) which is caused by FIP virus, a feline coronavirus. FIP-induced effusions are high in protein, mostly due to globulin (they characteristically coagulate like a jelly once exposed to air). Cellularity is usually high and mixed, to the extent this is regarded as an exudate but, importantly, no bacteria are observed, distinguishing

it from a septic exudate. Septic exudates also tend to be more opaque in comparison.

The image is a good example of the effusive or 'wet' form of FIP, although there is also a pyogranulomatous component (Fig. 3.5a, yellow circle). While the wet and dry forms classically represent two extremes of the disease spectrum, a mixed form occurs quite commonly, as here. FIP tends to occur in young, pure breed cats. Histopathology is generally confirmatory, especially when supported by immunohistochemistry directed against feline coronavirus antigen. Key organs to collect (for example, in a laparotomy) include liver, lymph node and kidney.

---

See also case RESP10.

---

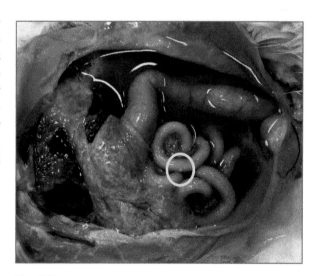

Fig. 3.5a

## References

1  Zachary, J. F. (Ed.) (2017). Mechanisms of microbial infections. In *Pathologic basis of veterinary disease* (6th ed). Elsevier. https://doi.org/10.1016/B978-0-323-35775-3.00004-7

2  Kennedy, M. A. (2020). Feline infectious peritonitis: Update on pathogenesis, diagnostics, and treatment. *Veterinary Clinics of North America. Small Animal Practice, 50*(5), 1001–1011. https://doi.org/10.1016/j.cvsm.2020.05.002

# GIT5 answers

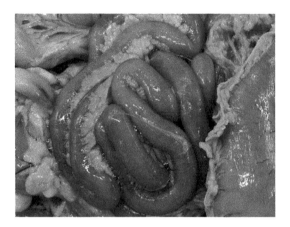

Fig. 3.6

## 1.  Describe any abnormalities

The lesions are subtle, but the small intestine is segmentally moderately dilated and slightly redder than normal (compare the slightly more normal loops in the top left of the image with those in the centre). There is scant, pale fawn membranous material (fibrin) on the serosal surface. The serosa is also very slightly granular ('ground glass' appearance).

## 2.  Provide a diagnosis

Moderate segmental acute enteropathy with fibrinous serositis.

This is a good, if subtle, example of canine parvovirus enteropathy. Classically, this virus causes crypt necrosis due to its requirement to infect rapidly dividing cells in order to survive and propagate. There is usually little inflammation, unless there is secondary infection. A helpful feature is loss of the normal velvety texture of the mucosal epithelium, which happens due to villous atrophy. In more severe cases, the intestinal content will be blood-tinged and malodorous with areas of erosion and ulceration. The gross appearance can range from segmental portions of intestine which are deep pink to crimson to dark red. As in this case, there may be very little colour change with, instead, a serosal 'ground glass' appearance, which may be due to subserosal oedema or serositis (the exact cause of this is uncertain).

## 3.  Provide some differential diagnoses for **acute** vomiting and diarrhoea in the adult dog

Table 3.1

| Vomiting | | Diarrhoea | |
|---|---|---|---|
| Infectious | Non-infectious | Infectious | Non-infectious |
| Not many! | Pyometra | Parvovirus | Food allergy |
| Parvovirus | Foreign body / obstruction | Parasites (*Giardia, Coccidia, Cryptosporidium, Trichuris, Taenia, etc.*) | Dietary indiscretion |
| | Gastric dilation and volvulus | Salmonella | Endocrine disease |
| | Intestinal torsion / volvulus / intussusception | | |
| | Toxin (e.g. dietary indiscretion, chocolate, drugs, ethylene glycol) | Campylobacter | |
| | Gastritis / gastric ulcer | Yersinia | |
| | Organic disease (e.g. pancreatitis, liver failure, acute renal failure, diabetic ketoacidosis) | Clostridium | |
| | Sepsis | Other* | |

Notes: *Rotavirus, coronavirus, *E. coli*, Shigella, among others. There are many potential causes of vomiting and diarrhoea in the dog, but many will have a chronic or intermittent presentation, rather than acute.[1]

## Reference

1   Elwood, C., Devauchelle, P., Elliott, J., Freiche, V., German, A. J., Gualtieri, M., Hall, E., Den Hertog, E., Neiger, R., Peeters, D., Roura, X., & Savary-Bataille, K. (2010). Emesis in dogs: A review. *Journal of Small Animal Practice*, 51(1), 4–22. https://doi.org/10.1111/j.1748-5827.2009.00820.x

# GIT6 answers

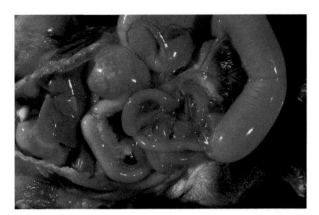

Fig. 3.7

## 1. Describe any abnormalities

The small intestine is focally replaced by a thin membrane for a distance of approximately 3 mm (see Fig. 3.7a). The small intestine proximal to this point is markedly distended and thin-walled (up to approximately 2.5 cm diameter). Distal to this point the diameter varies up to a maximum of ~1 cm diameter.

## 2. Provide a diagnosis

Segmental small intestinal atresia.

## 3. Define atresia and how it differs from stenosis; provide some possible causes of death in this case

Atresia means that there has been complete occlusion of the intestinal lumen due to failure of normal development of the tissue *in utero*. This can appear as a membrane, as in this case, but there are other subtypes.[1] These lesions are congenital and believed to have an ischaemic cause. The term stenosis denotes narrowing or incomplete obstruction of the intestine.

Intestinal obstruction leads to accumulation of ingesta and fluid from secretions originating from the stomach, pancreas, intestine and biliary tree. In this case, these secretions would have led to the marked segmental dilation of the small intestine. Upper gastrointestinal obstruction leads to vomiting, dehydration, hypokalaemia, hypochloraemia, and acid/base imbalance. Thus, death in these cases is likely due to an electrolyte imbalance or acid/base disturbances.

> Note: This case emphasises how important it is to thoroughly examine every body system in every case. This particular puppy was an end-of-week submission (late on a Friday) and it would have been easy to consider it as just another weak puppy with ill thrift. That is what we initially thought – we were quite surprised to find this lesion, a timely lesson that we cannot afford to be complacent. The intestinal dilation was a clear flag to 'follow the lesion' in this case, i.e. dilation in an otherwise well-preserved intestine can indicate obstruction, so always check for this.

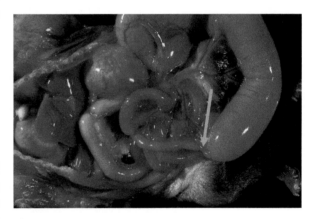

Fig. 3.7a

## Reference

1 Uzal, F. A., Plattner, B. L., & Hostetter, J. M. (2016). Alimentary system. In M. G. Maxie (Ed.), *Jubb, Kennedy and Palmer's pathology of domestic animals* (6th ed), Vol. 2. Elsevier. https://doi.org/10.1016/B978-0-7020-5318-4.00007-3

# GIT7 answers

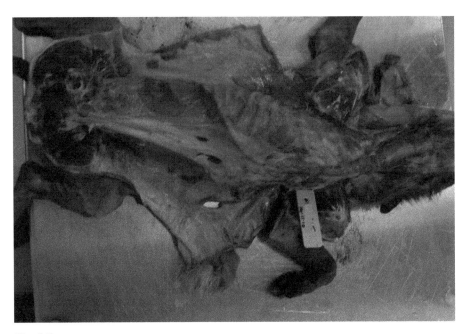

Fig. 3.8

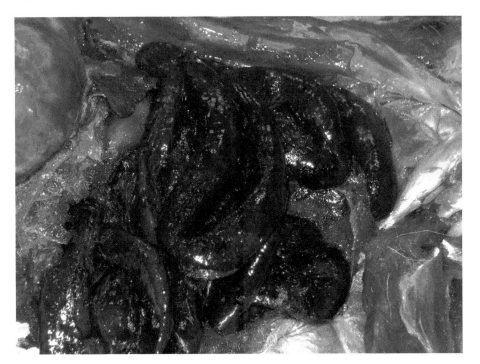

Fig. 3.9

## 1.   Describe any abnormalities

There is a generalised absence of peripheral fat reserves (and also internal peri-visceral fat, although this is more difficult to appreciate). The small intestine is diffusely dark purple, dilated and thin-walled. Particularly in Fig. 3.8, a marked reduction in muscle mass is also appreciable.

## 2.   Provide a diagnosis

a.  Emaciation and generalised muscle atrophy.
b.  Severe, diffuse, acute, small intestinal haemorrhage and necrosis (another acceptable gross diagnosis would be *severe diffuse acute haemorrhagic enteritis*).

### 3.  What is the most likely pathogenesis of the lesion in Fig. 3.9?

The lesion in Fig. 3.9 is most likely the result of mesenteric torsion. In mesenteric torsion, the small intestine rotates around the root of the mesentery (strictly speaking this is actually a volvulus as the twist is around the mesentery, rather than a torsion, where the twist is around the axis of the organ), but such is life with medical and veterinary terminology).* The twist compresses the vasculature supplying the intestine, causing ischaemia, haemorrhage and necrosis. Death would have been due to loss of mucosal integrity and bacteraemia / sepsis, exacerbated and likely preceded by hypovolaemia / lactic acidosis.

> Note: *Distinguishing torsion from volvulus is academic, since the end result is blockage of the blood supply, i.e. ischaemia, leading to hypoxia and necrosis. However, it is still important to be aware that there is a difference. An appropriate aetiological diagnosis is *ischaemic enteropathy*.

Reasonable differentials are haemorrhagic gastroenteritis and 'shock gut'. However, in the real-life situation where you can touch organs and examine them more fully (compared to an image), mesenteric torsion can usually be confirmed by passing your hand dorsally to the root of the mesentery and feeling for the twist site. The entire jejunum (duodenum and ileum perhaps less so) will usually be dark red and the colon spared, which can help to distinguish from shock gut.

> See also case GIT3.

### TIP: FREEZING

One additional thing we did not mention before, and that you may have noticed, is subtle white speckling over the serosal surface of the small intestine. There is also crystalline material on the omentum cranial to the intestine. The speckles and crystalline material are ice crystals. This dog had been frozen for some time prior to necropsy. This is not a diagnosis, however – it is an artefact, i.e. something that has been added after death that has nothing to do with the disease or cause of death (see CVS4 for the definition of artefact).

This case is a good example of how all is not always lost by freezing a body. A macroscopically dramatic lesion such as this will still be appreciable. Histopathology would have been significantly impacted but was not critical to the diagnosis in this event. Freezing is less likely to impact on trauma cases, for example, where fractured bones or large areas of haemorrhage will still be apparent. However, when considering whether or not to freeze a body prior to necropsy, the general rule of thumb is DO NOT – at least not if you can possibly avoid it. Freeze / thaw artefact leads to a catastrophic collection of artefacts. It will cause widespread haemolysis leading to red discolouration of soft tissues, such that contrast is lost, making it difficult to appreciate lesions, especially more subtle ones. The ice crystals also cause cell damage, to the extent that cell preservation is suboptimal (often significantly) and can hamper histological assessment, particularly in areas such as the intestinal tract, nervous system, renal tubules and liver. The best approach is to chill the body in a fridge. If chilled quickly, the body can remain in the fridge for a few days.

It is also worth noting that freezing can often negatively impact on bacterial culture so, if there is no option but to freeze, try to take samples for culture first. Freezing, happily, does not impact on toxicology. Samples suitable for toxicology can be collected at necropsy and frozen for storage and testing later, as needed. The same is largely true of samples collected for molecular testing, such as polymerase chain reaction (PCR).

# GIT8 answers

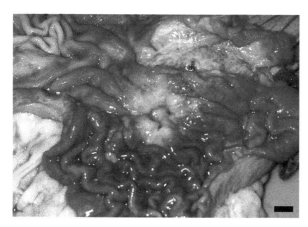

Fig. 3.10 **Bar = 1 cm.**

## 1.   Describe any abnormalities

There is a well-demarcated ('punched-out'), depressed area of mucosal loss in the fundus of the stomach, measuring approximately 1 cm diameter. It has a smooth, white (blanched), slightly contracted rim that measures approximately 0.75 cm thick circumferentially.

## 2.   Provide a diagnosis

Focal chronic gastric ulcer.

The blanched appearance around the ulcer corresponds to fibrosis – this would have felt firm grossly – and it indicates chronicity. Acute ulcers are often redder (perhaps with superimposed haemorrhage) and tend to have a more sharply demarcated, flat or flush edge. Figs 3.10a and b below depict an acute gastric ulcer with perforation, in which part of the wall is still intact.

Gastric ulcers carry the risk of perforation, in which case you may see signs of localised or generalised peritonitis (refer to the foreign body case in this section as presentation at necropsy may be similar in terms of the peritonitis).

## 3.   List **FOUR** possible causes of this lesion in the dog

a. Non-steroidal anti-inflammatory drugs (they inhibit bicarbonate secretion by reducing prostaglandin production – bicarbonate is important for maintaining a neutral ph at the gastric mucosal surface, as opposed to an acid pH in the lumen).

b. Stress.

c. Glucocorticoids.

d. Underlying neoplasia (gastric carcinoma; gastrinoma in the pancreas; mast cell tumour anywhere).

e. Liver disease – ulcers tend to be duodenal. Liver failure is believed to lead to reduced degradation of gastrin and histamine.[1]

f. Peptic ulcers occur but are not common.

g. Uraemia – can cause vasculitis and ischaemic necrosis of the mucosa but damage is usually microscopic.

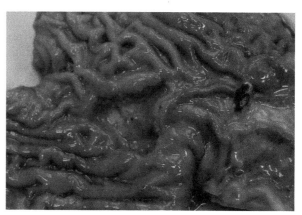

Fig. 3.10a

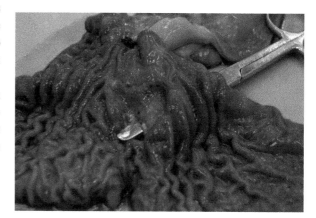

Fig. 3.10b

## Reference

1   Stanton, M. E., & Bright, R. M. (1989). Gastroduodenal ulceration in dogs. Retrospective study of 43 cases and literature review. *Journal of Veterinary Internal Medicine*, *3*(4), 238–244. https://doi.org/10.1111/j.1939-1676.1989.tb00863.x

# GIT9 answers

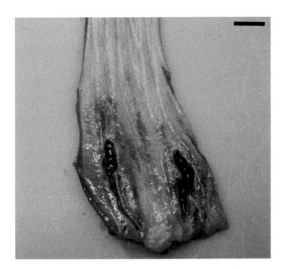

Fig. 3.11 Bar = 1 cm.

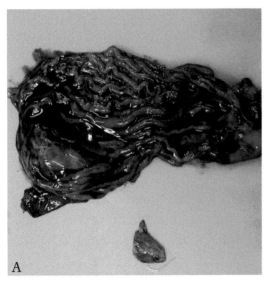

A

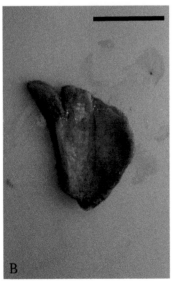

B

Fig. 3.12 A–B Bar = 1 cm.

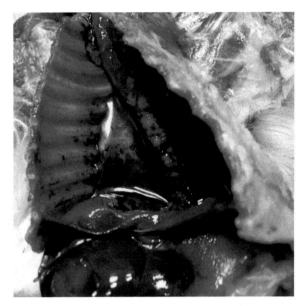

Fig. 3.13

## 1. Describe any abnormalities

Fig. 3.11: This is the opened oesophagus (longitudinally oriented linear ridges help to identify). On the mucosal surface there are two well-demarcated, linear, brown foci of mucosal loss, measuring up to 3–4 mm wide. The surrounding mucosal surface is mottled red/brown.

Fig 3.12A: This is the opened stomach which is empty other than a small amount of dark brown liquid. Adjacent to the stomach there is a solid, pale brown triangular foreign body.

Fig 3.12B: Higher magnification of the foreign body indicates it is a piece of bone that measures ~1.5 cm × 1.5 cm at its widest dimensions.

Fig 3.13. This is the opened thoracic cavity. It contains a small volume of dark red fluid which partially obscures multifocal to coalescing dark red foci on the parietal pleura that measure up to ~5 mm diameter.

NB: It is always best to evaluate cavity effusions prior to removing any organs, to avoid confounding with leakage of fluid from vessels, etc.

## 2. Provide a diagnosis/es

a. Multifocal subacute oesophageal ulcers (or tears) – oesophagus.
b. Intra-luminal haemorrhage and foreign body – stomach.
c. Mild haemothorax with acute petechial and ecchymotic haemorrhage – thoracic cavity.

### 3.    Provide a summary to explain the cause of death and pathogenesis of the findings in this dog

The bone foreign body caused the mucosal tears in the oesophagus, leading to haemorrhage. The oesophageal blood drained into the stomach accounting for the brown-tinged fluid on the gastric mucosal surface ('older' blood changes from red to chocolate brown as it is no longer oxidised). The haemothorax and petechial haemorrhage on the parietal surface of the thoracic cavity are indicators that this dog had likely gone into septic shock, leading to disseminated intravascular coagulopathy (DIC). This was likely due to the oesophageal damage, resulting in release of bacteria and their toxins into the blood stream. The initial pathogenesis of septic shock, and how it can lead to DIC, is summarised in case GIT2.

DIC is a life-threatening condition that occurs when the fine balance between pro-coagulants and anticoagulants is lost in favour of coagulation. Coagulation becomes uncontrolled and widespread (i.e. 'disseminated'). The widespread accumulation of intravascular fibrin (thrombosis) causes depletion of coagulation factors, known as consumptive coagulopathy. This leads to a propensity to bleed and, in this case, was the cause of the haemothorax as well as the petechial and ecchymotic haemorrhages. A number of different aetiologies can cause this imbalance, but sepsis is the most common. Others include cancer, severe tissue injury such as burns or heat stroke, and obstetric catastrophes.[1]

Regardless of the inciting cause, excessive tissue factor (TF) leads to overwhelming thrombin production that overcomes the body's natural inhibitors of thrombosis. As thrombin enhances platelet function, a vicious circle develops. The paradox is that haemorrhage is more likely as platelets, coagulation factors and fibrinogen are depleted by the previously mentioned overconsumption.

### Reference

1  Papageorgiou, C., Jourdi, G., Adjambri, E., Walborn, A., Patel, P., Fareed, J., Elalamy, I., Hoppensteadt, D., & Gerotziafas, G. T. (2018). Disseminated intravascular coagulation: An update on pathogenesis, diagnosis, and therapeutic strategies. *Clinical and Applied Thrombosis/Hemostasis, 24* (9S), 8S–28S. https://doi.org/10.1177/1076029618806424

# GIT10 answers

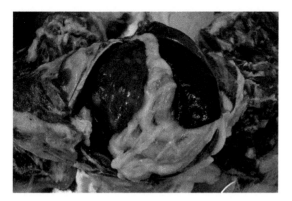

**Fig. 3.14**

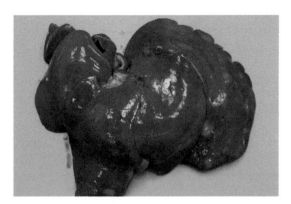

**Fig. 3.15**

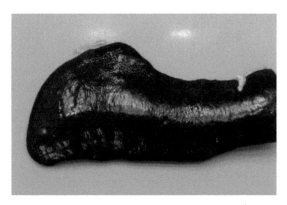

**Fig. 3.16**

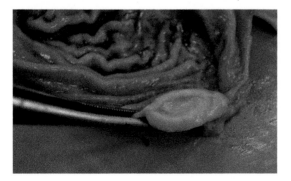

**Fig. 3.17**

## 1. Describe any abnormalities

Fig 3.14: Opened abdominal cavity with ventral aspect of three liver lobes, the spleen and the small intestine visible through the omentum. The liver lobes are diffusely tan (should be dark brown) and have rounded borders. The left lateral lobe in particular contains several, multifocally distributed, off-white nodules that range in diameter up to approximately 2 cm. The spleen is markedly enlarged and dark red/purple, with rounded borders.

Fig. 3.15: The liver is as described in Fig. 3.14, though the nodules affect other lobes.

Fig. 3.16: The spleen is as described in Fig. 3.14.

Fig. 3.17: There is a focal, ~3 cm × 1.5 cm × 1 cm, off-white, oval mass in the wall of the stomach.

## 2. Provide a diagnosis/es

a. Gastric carcinoma with metastases to the liver.
b. Moderate diffuse hepatopathy.
c. Marked splenomegaly.

## 3.

### a) Given the clinical history, explain the colour and size of the liver

The liver pallor and enlargement (as indicated by its rounded borders) may be due to fatty change (lipidosis) following prolonged inappetence but, given the history of steroid treatment, steroid hepatopathy is also possible (or both may be occurring at the same time).

### b) What is the clinical significance of the splenic changes?

This dog was euthanised so the enlarged spleen is likely due to barbiturate exposure, which leads to pooling of red blood cells in the spleen. It is a common necropsy finding that is not a true lesion, but a postmortem change.

### c) Provide some **non-neoplastic** differentials for the liver nodules

In general, the main differentials for *non-neoplastic* liver nodules are nodular hyperplasia and nodular regeneration. The former is more common in the older dog and has no clinical significance. On cut section, nodules of hyperplasia are usually a similar texture to the rest of the liver and non-compressive. They also tend to blend with the surrounding parenchyma. Nodular regeneration is a **clinically significant** lesion that occurs when there has been liver injury leading to hepatocellular loss. So, we would expect to see some liver scarring, perhaps an uneven capsular surface or a firm texture due to accompanying fibrosis. Nodular regeneration is a key part of cirrhosis, along with hepatocellular loss and fibrosis.

[In this case the hepatic nodules were due to metastatic carcinoma from the stomach so neoplasia is also always worth bearing in mind when faced with multiple nodular lesions in the liver].
    See also case HEP2.

## Further comment

Gastric carcinoma is not a common cancer in the dog, accounting for <1% of all canine tumours[1] and it may present as a mass protruding into the lumen, a mass within the wall, or as a crater-like lesion. It is a disease of the older animal and affected dogs present very much as this case did. Seventy to 90% of cases have developed metastases by the time the diagnosis is made, likely because clinical signs are often not appreciable in the early stages of the disease. The prognosis is poor. The most common metastatic sites are the regional lymph nodes, but the liver, lungs and spleen may be involved and other more unusual sites of spread include the duodenum, adrenal glands, pancreas and omentum.[1,2] The pylorus and lesser curvature of the stomach are mostly affected and, while the tumour in this case presented as a mass, they often extend transmurally and approximately half will manifest as an ulcer. An important gross feature diagnostically is the scirrhous reaction (fibrosis) that often accompanies this carcinoma, leading to increased firmness in the surrounding tissue. The cause of gastric carcinoma is not certain and likely to be multifactorial. Other possible neoplasms arising in the canine stomach include leiomyoma, leiomyosarcoma, carcinoid, lymphoma, mast cell tumour and gastrointestinal stromal tumour (GIST). GISTs are more common in the intestinal tract but can arise in the stomach.

## References

1   Hugen, S., Thomas, R. E., German, A. J., Burgener, I. A., & Mandigers, P. J. J. (2017). Gastric carcinoma in canines and humans, a review. *Veterinary and Comparative Oncology*, *15*(3), 692–705. https://doi.org/10.1111/vco.12249

2   Uzal, F. A., Plattner, B. L., & Hostetter, J. M. (2016). Alimentary system. In M. G. Maxie (Ed.), *Jubb, Kennedy and Palmer's pathology of domestic animals* (6th ed), Vol. 2 (pp. 101–102). Elsevier. https://doi.org/10.1016/B978-0-7020-5318-4.00007-3

# GIT11 answers

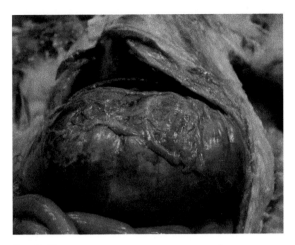

Fig. 3.18

## 1.   Describe any abnormalities
The stomach is markedly distended and the serosal surface is diffusely dark purple. The spleen is displaced cranially.

## 2.   Provide a diagnosis
Gastric dilatation and volvulus (GDV).

## 3.

### a)   Briefly describe what has happened to this stomach, i.e. outline the pathogenesis
Prior to addressing this question specifically, it is important to point out that, as you look down upon the normal opened canine abdomen (i.e. look upon its ventral surface), the greater curvature of the stomach should be on the left side of the dog, with the spleen curling around it, also on the left side. The pylorus, duodenum and pancreas are normally on the right side of the dog's abdomen.

In GDV, the stomach becomes distended with air, and the pylorus and duodenum move both cranially and ventrally over the body of the stomach. At this stage, the spleen and body of the stomach twist in a clockwise direction viewed caudal to the standing dog, such that the spleen moves towards the dorsal midline, although its position can vary with degree of volvulus. In a 180° twist, the ventral surface of the stomach becomes dorsally positioned and the dorsal surface is ventral (i.e. the stomach flips); see Fig. 3.18a. Some authors suggest that volvulus precedes distension but this is not proven; in addition, volvulus does not happen every time – the stomach may only be distended – but, when volvulus does occur, it leads to complete blockage of the gastro-oesophageal junction and eventual entrapment of the pylorus.

### b)   Provide some possible causes.
Suggested causes, or predisposing factors, are:[1]

- large breed dogs with deep chests, though any dog can be affected
- feeding one large meal a day
- using an elevated bowl
- ingestion of air
- stress
- lean body condition
- previous splenic disease
- increased laxity of the gastrosplenic ligament.

### c)   How might this lead to sudden death, as it did in this case?
The increased abdominal pressure leads to a reduction in venous return by compressing the caudal vena cava

⇩

Blood pools in vessels supplying the abdominal cavity

⇩

Hypovolaemia, ischaemia of the gastrointestinal tract, systemic hypotension and hypovolaemic shock

⇩

GI ischaemia leads to loss of mucosal integrity and endotoxaemia, leading to endotoxic shock and metabolic acidosis

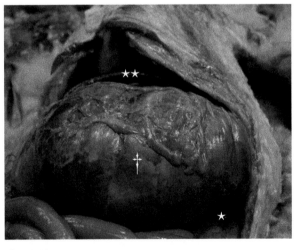

Fig. 3.18a

*The spleen should be here but the twisting of the stomach has dragged it 180° from its normal position to where it is now (**).

† While situated ventrally this is actually the dorsal surface of the gastric fundus. To correct this, you would need to place your widely spread hand over the visible surface of the stomach and rotate anticlockwise by 180°.

TIP

The twist could be more or less than 180° and, if 360°, you might be fooled into thinking it was in the correct position – but distension and discolouration are very helpful clues.

In any sudden death always check the stomach for distension early in the necropsy. Since gas distension can occur as a postmortem change (due to decomposition), and discolouration may become obscured with time after death, it is also important to feel for a twist at the gastro-oesophageal junction and pay attention to the location of the spleen. Once you start removing organs, it is too late.

## Reference

1    Uzal, F. A., Plattner, B. L., & Hostetter, J. M. (2016). Alimentary system. In M. G. Maxie (Ed.), *Jubb, Kennedy and Palmer's pathology of domestic animals* (6th ed), Vol. 2 (pp. 101–102). Elsevier. https://doi.org/10.1016/B978-0-7020-5318-4.00007-3

# GIT12 answers

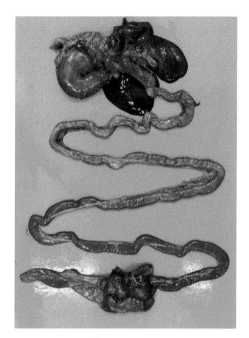

Fig. 3.19

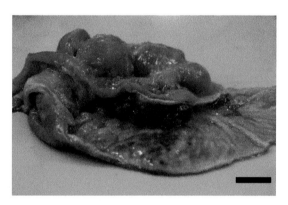

Fig. 3.20 Bar = 1 cm.

## 1. Describe any abnormalities in the images

The serosal surfaces are diffusely discoloured dark pink (freeze-thaw artefact). There is a focally extensive, multinodular mass at the ileocaeocolic junction, measuring up to 6 cm × 3 cm × 3 cm. Part of the mass extends into the lumen of the intestine, where it forms a dark brown to black, exophytic, botryoid but sessile nodule with associated black, elevated plaque-like areas. The lesion also involves/obscures the ileocaecocolic lymph nodes.

## 2. Provide a diagnosis

In a cat, lymphoma is the most likely cause of a gastrointestinal mass, particularly at this site. There are some other differentials that are equally valid, however. Given the location, feline gastrointestinal eosinophilic sclerosing fibroplasia (FGESF) may also be considered. FGESF

is typically seen in middle-aged cats and may present with gastrointestinal signs due to a mass effect which tends to occur at the pylorus or ileocaecocolic junction.[1-3] Other possible neoplasms include feline intestinal adenocarcinoma, feline intestinal mast cell tumour, large granular lymphoma, and leiomyosarcoma (in the dog a gastrointestinal stromal tumour may also be considered). Feline infectious peritonitis can also result in mass-like lesions in the intestine and local lymph nodes but, typically, multiple smaller satellite lesions will also be noted along the serosal surface of the intestines and there may be multi-organ involvement.

## 3. In addition to the focal lesion at the ileocaecocolic junction, this cat also had multifocal, white, bulging nodules within the renal parenchyma but no other lesions were macroscopically appreciable. What is the most likely final diagnosis?

Given the involvement of the kidneys, feline intestinal lymphoma is the most likely final diagnosis in this case as this is the most common neoplastic process in the intestine of cats. Feline intestinal adenocarcinoma and mast cell tumours may also metastasise to other organs; cytological evaluation of impression smears from the lesions may be beneficial in differentiating the lesions but histological evaluation would be preferable. FGESF is an idiopathic and non-neoplastic condition that involves the gastrointestinal tract and local lymph nodes; spread to other organs is not reported (although there may be eosinophils detected in the circulation or other tissues).[1-3]

## References

1 Craig, L. E., Hardam, E. E., Hertzke, D. M., Flatland, B., Rohrbach, B. W., & Moore, R. R. (2009) Feline gastrointestinal eosinophilic sclerosing fibroplasia. *Veterinary Pathology*, 46(1), 63–70. https://doi.org/10.1354/vp.46-1-63

2 Sihvo, H. K., Simola, O. T., Vainionpää, M. H., & Syrjä, P. E. (2011). Pathology in practice. Severe chronic multifocal intramural fibrosing and eosinophilic enteritis, with occasional intralesional bacteria, consistent with feline gastrointestinal eosinophilic sclerosing fibroplasia. (FIESF). *Journal of the American Veterinary Medical Association*, 238(5), 585–587. https://doi.org/10.2460/javma.238.5.585

3 Linton, M., Nimmo, J. S., Norris, J. M., Churcher, R., Haynes, S., Zoltowska, A., Hughes, S., Lessels, N. S., Wright, M., & Malik, R. (2015). Feline gastrointestinal eosinophilic sclerosing fibroplasia: 13 cases and review of an emerging clinical entity. *Journal of Feline Medicine and Surgery*, 17(5), 392–404. https://doi.org/10.1177/1098612X14568170

# Respiratory cases

4

# RESP1

## Topics

**Lesion recognition**

**Generation of pathological differential diagnoses lists**

## History

A 9Y old, female neutered West Highland White Terrier died within 24 hours of developing sudden onset dyspnoea. There was a vague history of previous episodes of dyspnoea that resolved with antimicrobial therapy. Pertinent necropsy findings were a moderate sanguineous pleural effusion and lungs (depicted in Fig. 4.1) which were wet and heavy. The heart was grossly normal and there was no evidence of pulmonary thromboembolism.

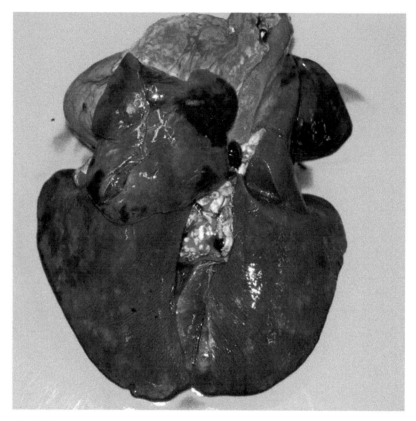

Fig. 4.1

## Questions

1. Describe any abnormalities.
2. Provide a diagnosis.
3. What causes might you consider for this case?

# RESP2

## Topics

Lesion recognition

Prioritisation of findings

Common artefacts and pitfalls

## History

A 3Y old, male neutered domestic longhair cat was found dead in the owner's kitchen, having been completely normal earlier that morning. The only gross abnormality is shown in Figs 4.2 and 4.3.

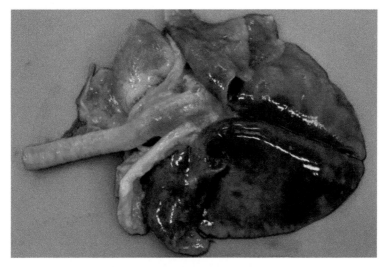

Fig. 4.2   Image credit: Dr David Walker.

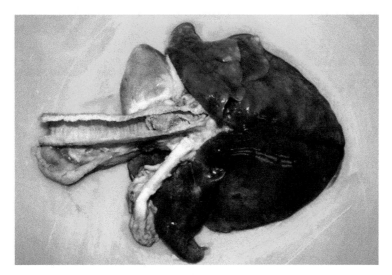

Fig. 4.3   Image credit: Dr David Walker.

## Questions

1. Describe any abnormalities.
2. Provide a diagnosis.
3. How significant is this lesion?

# RESP3

## Topics

Lesion recognition

Pathogenesis

## History

Review Fig. 4.4, which illustrates the findings in the thoracic cavity of a 5Y old, male Ragdoll cat that presented for necropsy after a period of medically managed respiratory distress. Following clinical deterioration, the decision was made to euthanise the cat.

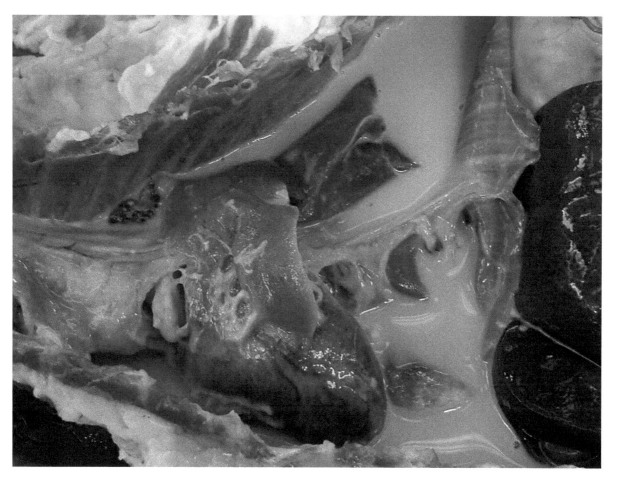

Fig. 4.4

## Questions

1. Describe any abnormalities.
2. Provide a diagnosis.
3. What other organs would you be interested in examining to help determine a cause?

# RESP4

## Topics

Lesion recognition

Generation of pathological differential diagnoses lists

## History

A 13Y old, female domestic shorthair cat presented with weight loss and recent respiratory distress that deteriorated in the face of symptomatic therapy. Radiographs indicated multiple lung masses and the owner elected for euthanasia. The lungs were removed at necropsy and are illustrated in Fig. 4.5. A cytological smear from one of the nodules, stained with Giemsa, is illustrated in Fig. 4.6.

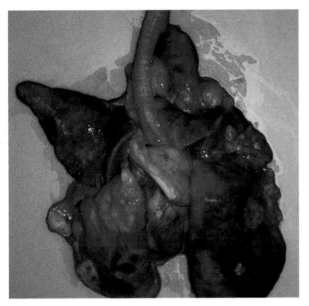

Fig. 4.5

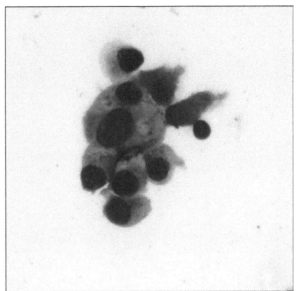

Fig. 4.6

## Questions

1. Describe any abnormalities.
2. Provide a diagnosis.
3. Justify your diagnosis and list some differentials.

# RESP5

## Topics

Lesion recognition

Generation of pathological differential diagnoses lists

Practical technique

## History

A 7Y old, male neutered Rough Collie presented with progressive stertor and a cough that did not respond to antimicrobial therapy. Due to deterioration, euthanasia was the ultimate outcome and a necropsy was performed. The most pertinent finding is highlighted in Figs 4.7 and 4.8.

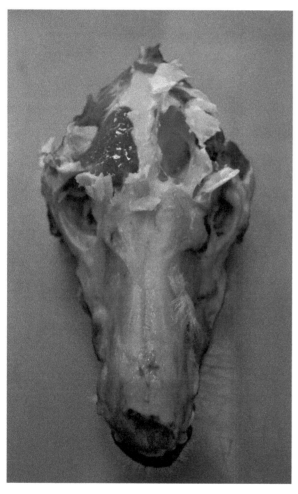

Fig. 4.7

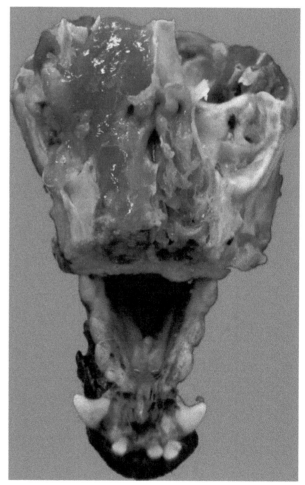

Fig. 4.8

## Questions

1. Describe any abnormalities.
2. Provide a diagnosis.
3. Outline how you would handle this sample to maximise the chances of a diagnosis?

# RESP6

## Topic

**Lesion recognition**

## History

Fig. 4.9 shows the lungs from an 11Y old, male Bulldog which died following a 2 day period of respiratory distress.

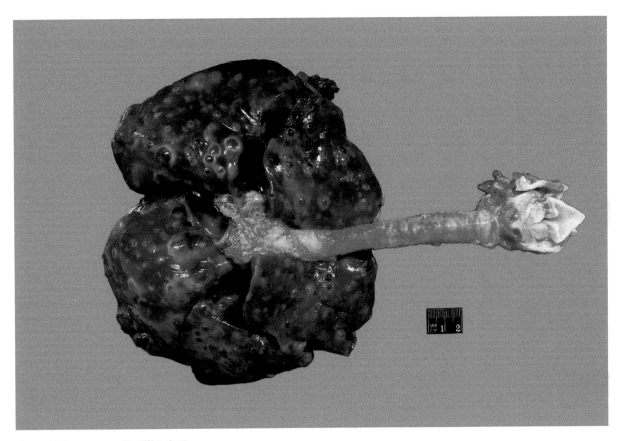

**Fig. 4.9** Image credit: Alistair Cox.

## Questions

1. Describe any abnormalities.
2. Provide a diagnosis.
3. Which other organ(s) would you be most interested in assessing?

# RESP7

**Lesion recognition**

**Prioritisation of findings**

## History

Necropsy finding in a 9Y old, male Chihuahua that had been euthanised following a road traffic accident and submitted for necropsy for insurance reasons.

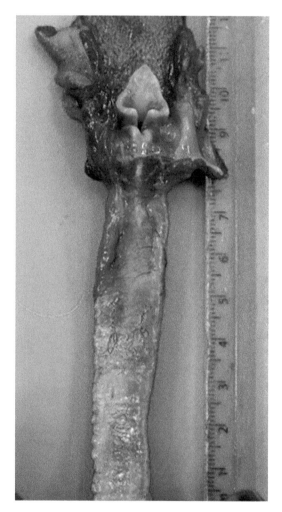

Fig. 4.10

## Questions

1. Describe any abnormalities.
2. Provide a diagnosis.
3. What is the cause of this lesion?

# RESP8

## Topics

Lesion recognition

Practical technique

## History

Necropsy findings in an 11Y old, male Terrier crossbreed dog with a history of chronic coughing progressing to dyspnoea, weight loss, anorexia and lethargy. The main lesion found at necropsy is shown in Fig. 4.11 (nudge: right side). There were no other gross findings.

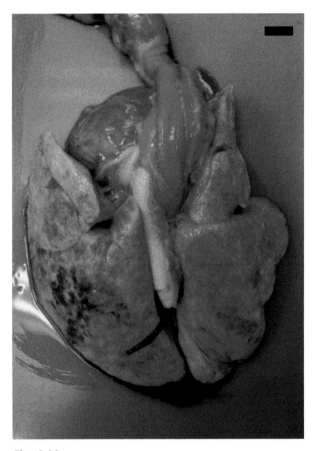

Fig. 4.11

## Questions

1. Describe any abnormalities.
2. Provide a diagnosis.
3. Which particular gross features tend to support your diagnosis?

# RESP9

## Topics

Lesion recognition

Generation of pathological differential diagnoses lists

Pathogenesis

## History

A 3Y old, female domestic shorthair cat died following a short illness characterised by respiratory distress (tachypnoea, open-mouthed breathing), pyrexia and anorexia. Radiographs had indicated a pattern consistent with fluid within the thoracic cavity and there was no response to supportive therapy. A necropsy was pursued as there were other in-contact cats in the home. The most important gross findings are illustrated in Fig. 4.12.

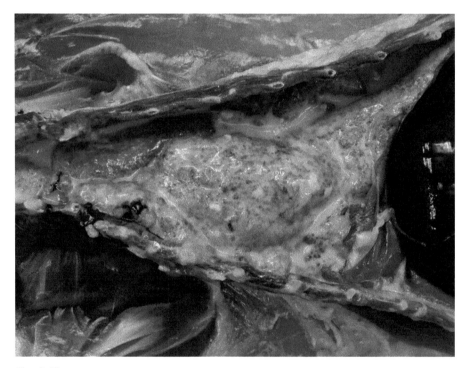

Fig. 4.12

## Questions

1. Describe any abnormalities.
2. Provide a diagnosis.
3. Briefly outline:
   a) a likely aetiology
   b) a potential pathogenesis
   c) **THREE** potential differentials based on the signalment and clinical history.

# RESP10

## Topics

Lesion recognition

Generation of pathological differential diagnoses lists

## History

A 6-month-old, male entire Bengal cat presented for necropsy following a prolonged history of inappetance, weight loss and variable pyrexia. Prior to euthanasia it was reported to have developed neurological signs. In the image below, tissue samples had been taken from the left caudal lung lobe for further testing prior to fixation. A smaller number of morphologically similar lesions were also noted on the epicardial surface of the left ventricle, meninges and rarely on the serosal surface of the gastrointestinal tract (Fig. 4.14).

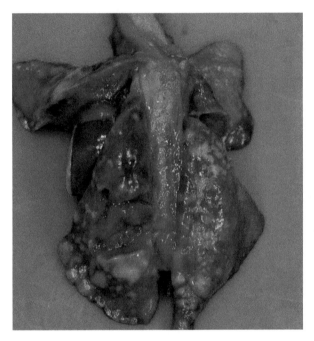

Fig. 4.13

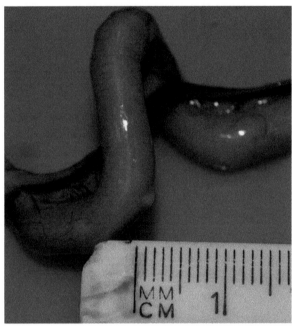

Fig. 4.14

## Questions

1. Describe any abnormalities.
2. Provide a morphological diagnosis for each image.
3. What causes might you consider for this case?

# RESP11

## Topics

Lesion recognition

Generation of pathological differential diagnoses lists

## History

A 12Y old, male neutered domestic short-haired cat was presented with a short history of lethargy, coughing and hyporexia. Chest X-rays showed a diffuse interstitial pattern in the lungs, with scattered ill-defined nodules. The cat deteriorated and the owners opted for euthanasia and necropsy. The lungs are show in Fig. 4.15 below.

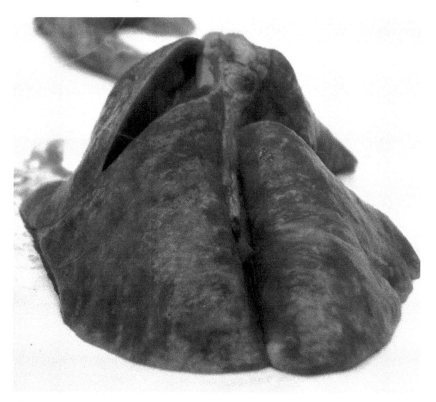

Fig. 4.15

## Questions

1. Describe any abnormalities.
2. Provide a morphological diagnosis.
3. What causes might you consider for this case?

# RESP1 answers

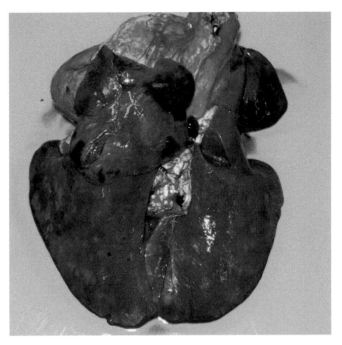

Fig. 4.1

## 1. Describe any abnormalities

All lung lobes are diffusely dark red. A slightly more subtle change is that they are not flaccid in that they do not spread out onto the table as normal lungs would. They tend to 'stand proud' because they are firmer than normal. These lungs would have a rubbery consistency if you could palpate them.

Note: The red discolouration also extended into the parenchyma on cut section.

## 2. Provide a diagnosis

This is compatible with interstitial pneumonia although histopathology would be required to rule out diffuse haemorrhage, which would appear similar. Bronchopneumonia would mainly affect the cranial lung lobes and the cranioventral aspects of the caudal lung lobes. Aspiration pneumonia tends to affect the right middle lung lobe or at least present as a lobar pneumonia (i.e. not diffuse). Embolic pneumonia is generally multifocal. Bronchointerstitial pneumonia affecting all lung lobes is possible but, strictly speaking, is a histological diagnosis as it targets a specific part of the lung. The morphological diagnosis in this case was: *Severe diffuse acute bilateral haemorrhagic interstitial pneumonia.* Interstitial pneumonia is quite a broad diagnosis which describes damage to, or inflammation of, the alveolar walls and interlobular septa. It requires histological confirmation. Type II pneumocyte hyperplasia, a reparative response, can

occur from around three days following insult but was not observed in this case (too acute).

## 3. What causes might you consider for this case?

There are many potential causes of acute interstitial pneumonia. However, necrosis and suppurative inflammation in this case raised the strong suspicion of a primary bacterial cause. *Streptococcus zooepidemicus* was a consideration and a sample of lung was submitted for bacterial culture. A heavy pure growth of *Escherichia coli* was isolated. Typing was not pursued but the histological lesions correlated well with those reported for necrotoxigenic *E. coli* in the dog. This strain expresses several virulence factors and has been identified as a cause of haemorrhagic pneumonia, vasculitis and thrombosis.[1] *Bordetella bronchiseptica* can also cause necrotising and haemorrhagic pneumonia in the dog but is generally more regional, affecting individual lobes. It is also more common in puppies.

Other differentials for acute interstitial pneumonia in dogs include canine distemper, canid herpesvirus 1 (neonates), *Pasteurella multocida, Klebsiella pneumoniae* and, less commonly, canine influenza. Canine adenovirus type 2 causes bronchointerstitial pneumonia so would be a reasonable gross differential in this case. Paraquat toxicosis and underlying uraemia are also worth considering, as is diffuse alveolar damage following sepsis, endotoxaemia or shock, so-called acute respiratory distress syndrome (ARDS) or 'shock lung'. West Highland White Terriers are predisposed to interstitial fibrosis, but this would present progressively over a longer period and, while the lungs are usually diffusely affected and firm, they are not usually red. Widespread interstitial collagen deposition is a key histological feature.[2]

Helpful historical features in cases like this include vaccination and worming history; any medical treatment or potential exposure to drugs or toxins (especially those with anticoagulant properties); any previous or current underlying illnesses, if known; presence of pyrexia; or clinical signs such as vomiting.

---

TIP

The pleural surface of the lungs may become red due to exposure to the environment. It is therefore important to serially section the lung to ensure any redness extends into the parenchyma, in which case it is more likely to be significant.

Lung that sinks in water is abnormal – this may indicate atelectasis (collapse), inflammation (pneumonia) and/or haemorrhage, though not usually oedema.

Remember that hypostatic ('downside') congestion will generally lead to unilateral and diffuse red discolouration that extends into the parenchyma; however, affected lung will float, assuming it is otherwise normal.

---

## References

1 Breitschwerdt, E. B., DebRoy, C., Mexas, A. M., Brown, T. T., & Remick, A. K. (2005). Isolation of necrotoxigenic *Escherichia coli* from a dog with hemorrhagic pneumonia. *Journal of the American Veterinary Medical Association, 226*(12), 2016–2019. https://doi.org/10.2460/javma.2005.226.2016

2 Laurila, H. P., & Rajamäki, M. M. (2020). Update on canine idiopathic pulmonary fibrosis in West Highland white terriers. *Veterinary Clinics of North America. Small Animal Practice, 50*(2), 431–446. https://doi.org/10.1016/j.cvsm.2019.11.004

# RESP2 answers

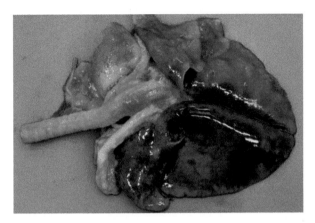

Fig. 4.2

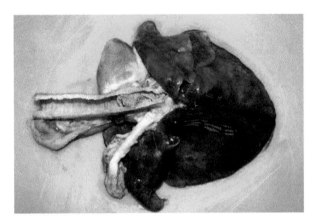

Fig. 4.3

## 1.   Describe any abnormalities

In Fig. 4.2, there is slight pale brown discolouration and distension of the trachea, just cranial to the tracheal bifurcation. Fig. 4.3 shows that the tracheal lumen in this area is filled with a pellet of soft, fawn material. This material is aspirated food, which had occluded the tracheal lumen and the most cranial aspect of both main stem bronchi (the latter not visible in the images). This would have led to obstruction, asphyxiation and death. The left lung lobes are diffusely dark red, compatible with hypostatic congestion, an insignificant postmortem artefact due to pooling of blood on the downside of the animal.

## 2.   Provide a diagnosis

Intra-luminal tracheal foreign body with obstruction.

## 3.   How significant is this lesion?

Highly significant as it is the cause of death. It would have resulted in asphyxiation and it correlated with the acute nature of this cat's death. In this case, there had been the suspicion of toxin exposure and it was potentially feasible that something toxic had triggered vomiting, predisposing the cat to aspiration of food material. However, there was nothing to suggest toxin exposure grossly, such as haemorrhage (e.g. due to rodenticide exposure), abnormal material in the stomach, or abnormal visceral organs. Histopathology did not identify any toxic change in major visceral organs (e.g. no evidence of ethylene glycol toxicity, nephrotoxicity or hepatotoxicity). There was also no evidence of trauma, infection, neoplasia or congenital disease and samples of stomach content, liver and kidney were negative for toxins (broad panel). Other conditions that were considered and ruled out in this case were a cardiomyopathy, particularly given the young age, and pulmonary artery thromboembolism, which is a cause of sudden death in dogs and cats.

This case highlights how, even in the face of finding a significant lesion (blockage of the trachea) which would explain unexpected death, it is still wise to collect further samples suitable for toxicology, in case there are queries over how or why the lesion occurred that may ultimately require further investigation.

# RESP3 answers

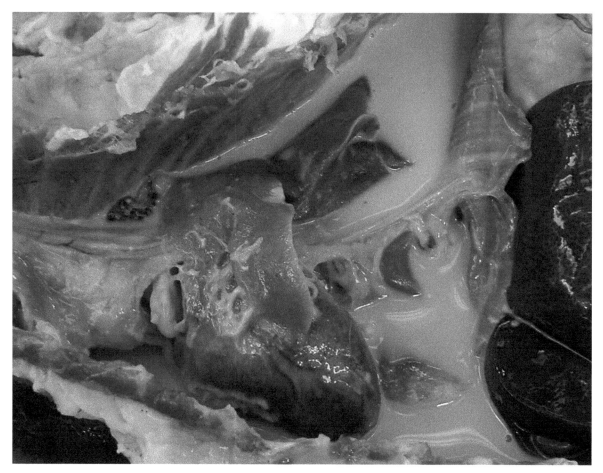

Fig. 4.4

## 1.   Describe any abnormalities

The thoracic cavity contains a moderate to large amount of opaque, pink fluid. The lung lobes are reduced in size (collapsed). There are deposits of pale yellow material on the pleural surface of the lungs and on the epicardial surface of the heart (fibrin).

## 2.   Provide a diagnosis

Severe chylothorax with marked diffuse pulmonary atelectasis.

## 3.   What other organs would you be interested in examining to help determine a cause?

The heart is particularly important since chylothorax is a potential consequence of hypertrophic cardiomyopathy. Other causes include idiopathic chylothorax, obstruction of lymphatic drainage (by a neoplastic or inflammatory intrathoracic mass) or thoracic duct rupture (actually uncommon although frequently cited as a likely cause). As an aside, the fluid mainly comprises small mature lymphocytes, although there may be smaller numbers of macrophages admixed and, depending on chronicity, small numbers of neutrophils may also be present. The fibrin over the pleura and epicardium is likely due to the local irritation of the pleural surface by the chylous effusion.

---

TIP

Other abnormal intrathoracic accumulations that can cause diffuse pulmonary atelectasis include blood (haemothorax), serous fluid (hydrothorax), pus (pyothorax) and air (pneumothorax).

See also case RESP9.

# RESP4 answers

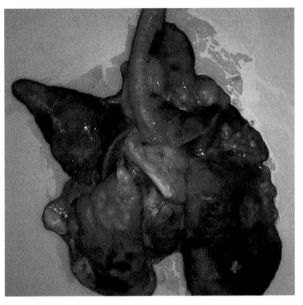

Fig. 4.5

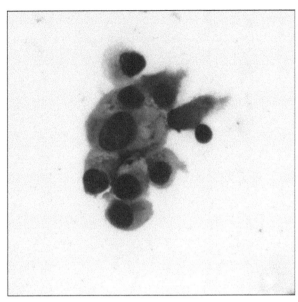

Fig. 4.6

## 1.  Describe any abnormalities

Fig. 4.5: There are multiple (at least seven) firm, raised, often coalescing masses scattered throughout all visible lung lobes, ranging in diameter from approximately 2–5 cm. Most are pale fawn/cream, multilobulated and well-demarcated with a smooth, shiny surface. Some are centrally depressed ('umbilicated').

Fig. 4.6: This smear comprises a cohesive cluster of atypical epithelial cells in which there are features of malignancy (marked anisocytosis, moderate to marked anisokaryosis, most nuclei contain at least one large nucleolus). Faint cilia are evident on a few of the cells.

## 2.  Provide a diagnosis

Pulmonary carcinoma with intra-pulmonary metastasis is most likely.

## 3.  Justify your diagnosis and list some differentials

The distribution of the pulmonary masses is typical of a metastatic pattern. Carcinoma deposits are often umbilicated, as in this case, and the cohesive, ciliated cells on cytology add further support to epithelial origin. The ciliation suggests this is most likely of primary pulmonary origin with subsequent metastasis to the lungs (the largest mass may be the primary). In the absence of ciliation and without knowledge of other necropsy findings, alternative primary epithelial tumours would have to be considered, such as mammary, cholangiocellular, gastrointestinal, pancreatic, thyroid, adrenal, mammary (in a female animal) and prostatic (in a male animal), among others.

# RESP5 answers

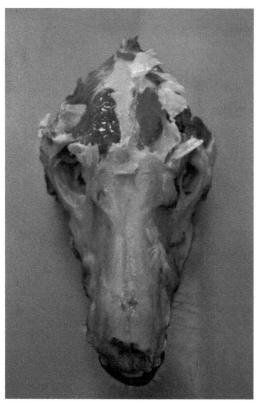

Fig. 4.7

Fig. 4.8

## 1.   Describe any abnormalities

The right frontal sinus is completely filled with semi-transparent, pale amber, gelatinous material.

## 2.   Provide a diagnosis

Mucinous adenocarcinoma is the most likely diagnosis. A large, cystic lesion is another potential differential.

## 3.   Outline how you would handle this sample to maximise the chances of a diagnosis?

a.  Fix a portion of the soft gelatinous material in 10% neutral buffered formalin.
b.  Serially section the sinus and surrounding calvaria to create slabs of bone for fixation and to further investigate the extent and character of the lesion. Fig. 4.8a illustrates how the lesion has a different morphological appearance in the maxillary bone proximal to the sinus. It consists of a non-encapsulated, pink, soft (but solid) mass that invades and replaces the maxillary bone. This area would be the best region for histopathology but would require decalcification. If available, a diamond saw would

help to cut thinner sections (~10 mm thick) prior to decalcification. The diamond saw and decalcification steps are usually undertaken by specialist histopathology laboratories, but thick, transverse slabs of bone could be collected 'in the field' using a good quality hacksaw and a new blade.
c.  It may also be worth collecting a portion of the gelatinous material for culture (to exclude fungal infection more confidently, for example).

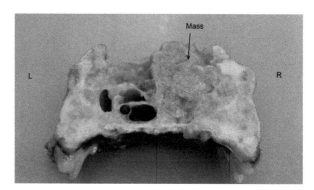

Fig. 4.8a

# RESP6 answers

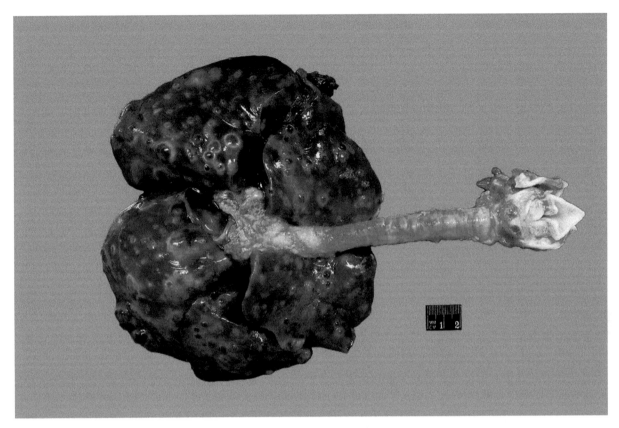

Fig. 4.9

## 1.  Describe any abnormalities

Disseminated throughout all visible lung lobes are multiple (innumerable), raised, smooth, shiny, translucent, red/grey nodules, many of which have a tan rim. The nodules range in diameter from approximately 1–10 mm. The intervening lung parenchyma is dark red (congested).

## 2.  Provide a diagnosis

This is most likely metastatic haemangiosarcoma. The translucent red appearance of the nodules is very characteristic of haemangiosarcoma (on cut section, the nodules appear cavitated and blood-filled). This would at least be the primary rule out. The multifocal (coalescing) distribution is consistent with secondary embolic spread (i.e. metastasis) which, in sarcomas, is typically via the haematogenous route.

## 3.  Which other organ(s) would you be most interested in assessing?

Right atrium of the heart, liver, spleen, skin and kidney are the most common primary sites to consider and check during necropsy.

# RESP7 answers

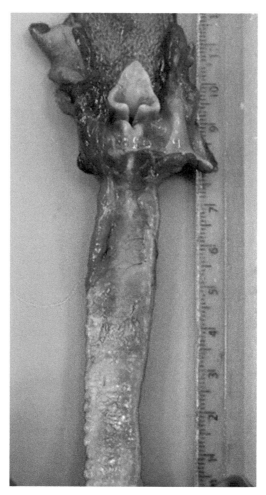

Fig. 4.10

### 1.   Describe any abnormalities

The tracheal ligament is wider than normal, measuring up to ~1.5 cm for almost the entire length of the trachea. As a result, there is dorsoventral flattening of the trachea.

### 2.   Provide a diagnosis

Tracheal collapse (or dysplasia).

### 3.   What is the cause of this lesion?

Tracheal collapse can be congenital or acquired. Congenital forms are due to abnormal glycoproteins in the cartilage rings, leading to softening. Acquired forms arise subse-quently to trauma, inflammation around the trachea, compressive masses or for iatrogenic reasons (e.g. tracheal intubation).[1] While it is most common in toy and minia-ture breeds, and may result in respiratory signs, it may also be an incidental finding at necropsy.

### Reference

1   Della Maggiore, A. (2020). An update on tracheal and airway collapse in dogs. *Veterinary Clinics of North America. Small Animal Practice*, 50(2), 419–430. https://doi.org/10.1016/j.cvsm.2019.11.003

# RESP8 answers

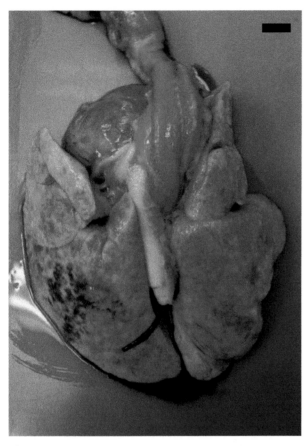

Fig. 4.11 **Bar = 1 cm.**

## 1.    Describe any abnormalities

Fig. 4.12 includes the lungs, heart, trachea, oesophagus and thoracic aorta. The most pertinent lesion is in the right caudal lung lobe. This lesion is ill-defined but measures approximately 2–3 cm diameter and has a contracted border with a central depressed, umbilicated pleural surface. The surrounding parenchyma is yellow, speckled and slightly raised (Fig. 4.11a). There is also an ill-defined, dark red, mottled lesion on the pleural surface of the left caudal lung lobe, measuring an area spanning approximately 6 cm.

## 2.    Provide a diagnosis

  a.  Pulmonary carcinoma – right caudal lung lobe.
  b.  Moderate, multifocal to coalescing, acute, ecchymotic pleural haemorrhage – left caudal lung lobe.

## 3.    Which particular gross features tend to support your diagnosis?

Confirmation would, of course, require histological evaluation but some features in the image and history support pulmonary carcinoma as the most likely gross diagnosis. The lesion is solitary, i.e. the pattern is not that of haematogenous or lymphatic spread from another primary site. It is possible that this is the first metastatic deposit to the lungs but that is less likely, given the lesion's size. The history also specifies that there were no other gross lesions. The umbilicated shape of the lesion and its contracted border are very suggestive of a carcinoma. The umbilication is likely due to central necrosis and the contracted border is due to a scirrhous reaction (fibroplasia and fibrosis as a response to the neoplasm). Even if there were multiple deposits, that would not rule out a primary pulmonary carcinoma as pulmonary carcinoma can metastasise to other lung lobes. However, at necropsy other potential primary sites would need to be ruled out, such as mammary gland, prostate gland, pancreas, gastrointestinal, anal sac, liver, thyroid gland, adrenal gland, kidney and skin, among others. The haemorrhage in the left caudal lung lobe is possibly an agonal change.

## Comment

Pulmonary carcinoma is actually quite a broad term denoting a malignant epithelial neoplasm arising in the lung. However, potential origins include the bronchial, bronchiolar or alveolar epithelium so there are several different subtypes. Some attempts have also been made to grade pulmonary carcinomas based on histological features.[1,2] The terms 'carcinoma' and 'adenocarcinoma' can be confusing to the novice. Both imply malignant epithelial neoplasia but 'adenocarcinoma' usually indicates that the neoplastic cells form *glandular* structures (i.e. acini), which can be helpful in further defining the possible origin. The term 'carcinoma' is more general or broad and can be used for tumours in which a glandular pattern is present but also in more solid epithelial malignancies or in those where nests, islands or trabeculae predominate (e.g. surface epithelial malignancies such as squamous cell carcinoma).

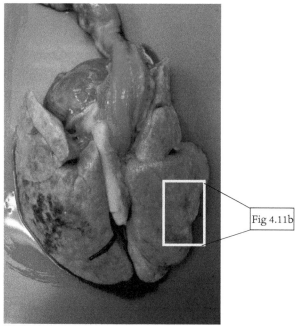

Fig. 4.11a

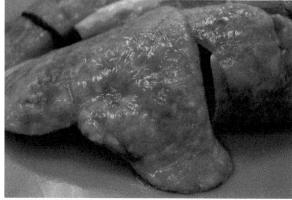

Fig. 4.11b

## TIP

- Examine organ externally then serially section.
- Sample a portion of tissue that is no thicker than a pencil (1 cm); as a guide, the other two dimensions should ideally measure 4–6 cm.
- Lung samples should include a grossly visible airway and pleural surface, i.e. do not just snip off the apex of a lobe.
- Sample multiple lobes (at least four).
- Only then can you safely palpate the lungs without inflicting artefact!
- Sample any other palpably abnormal areas.

## References

1   McNiel, E. A., Ogilvie, G. K., Powers, B. E., Hutchison, J. M., Salman, M. D., & Withrow, S. J. (1997). Evaluation of prognostic factors for dogs with primary lung tumors: 67 cases (1985–1992). *Journal of the American Veterinary Medical Association, 211*(11), 1422–1427.

2   Lee, B. M., Clarke, D., Watson, M., & Laver, T. (2020). Retrospective evaluation of a modified human lung cancer stage classification in dogs with surgically excised primary pulmonary carcinomas. *Veterinary and Comparative Oncology, 18*(4), 590–598. https://doi.org/10.1111/vco.12582

# RESP9 answers

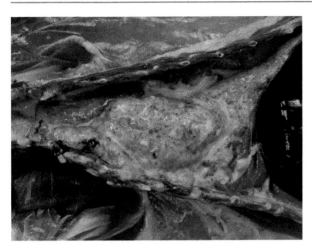

Fig. 4.12

## 1.  Describe any abnormalities

The thoracic organs are obscured, and the thoracic cavity is filled with opaque, white fluid containing small amounts of particulate material.

## 2.  Provide a diagnosis

Severe pyothorax.

## 3.  Briefly outline

### a)  A likely aetiology

This is most likely a bacterial infection given that the exudate is suppurative (bacterial cases are often mixed and of oral origin but other reported causes include *Staphylococcus, Streptococcus, E. coli, Nocardia, Actinomyces* and even *Salmonella* spp.).

### b)  A potential pathogenesis

Bacteria could achieve entry to the thoracic cavity by a number of routes: (i) direct inoculation via a traumatic wound (e.g. bite perforating the chest wall); (ii) rupture of oesophagus; (iii) extension from an abscess (e.g. lung lobe); (iv) haematogenous spread of bacterial infection to pleura or mediastinum; and (v) migrating foreign body.

### c)  THREE potential differentials based on the signalment and clinical history.

Main differentials for fluid in the thoracic cavity are outlined in Table 4.1.

Table 4.1 Differentials for fluid in the thoracic cavity.

| Type of fluid | Condition | Potential causes |
| --- | --- | --- |
| Blood | Haemothorax | Trauma; coagulopathy; neoplasia |
| Serous | Hydrothorax | Increased hydrostatic pressure (e.g. heart failure); reduced oncotic pressure (e.g. hypoproteinaemia); increased vascular permeability (e.g. vasculitis). |
| | | Feline infectious peritonitis would fall into this category, though often there is a high protein component to the fluid due to increased fibrin – such fluid has a tendency to partially solidify after exposure to air, turning to a gelatinous fluid or jelly. |
| Blood-tinged serous fluid | Serosanguineous effusion | Causes are similar to those outlined in the serous category above. |
| Chylous | Chylothorax | Defined as a fluid that is low in protein but high in lymphocytes – usually also opaque (like pus) but tends to be more 'milky' and pink-tinged. |
| Purulent | Pyothorax | The fluid present may vary in consistency and colour but is often off-white to yellow. The possible causes are outlined above. Submission of a sample for microbiology may yield a single organism but mixed infections also occur. |

# RESP10 answers

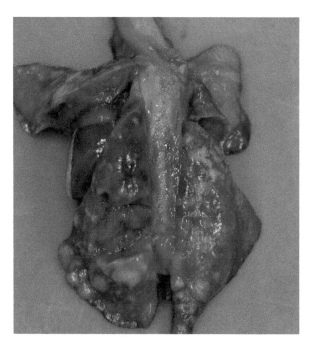

Fig. 4.13

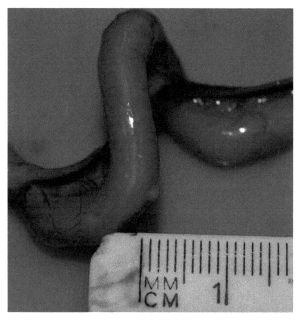

Fig. 4.14

### 1.   Describe any abnormalities

There are multifocal to coalescing, off-white nodules and plaques over the pleural surface of the lungs, ranging from <1–10 mm diameter and extending 2–4 mm into the underlying parenchyma.

There is a focal, 1 mm, raised, off-white nodule on the serosal surface of the small intestine.

### 2.   Provide a diagnosis.

   a. Severe, multifocal to coalescing pyogranulomatous pleuritis and pneumonia – lungs.

   b. Mild, focal, pyogranulomatous serositis – small intestine.

### 3.   Given the clinical history and other reported findings, what is the most likely final diagnosis in this case?

Given the clinical history of the patient and other reported changes, feline infectious peritonitis ('dry' form) would be the most likely cause. Feline infectious peritonitis (FIP) is caused by a mutation in feline enteric coronavirus that enables persistent infection of macrophages.[1,2] The diagnosis and management of FIP in cats is evolving but the 'gold standard' test is still considered to be histopathology with identification of characteristic lesions (vasculitis and pyogranulomatous inflammation) with immunohistochemical detection of feline coronavirus antigen within macrophages in the sections.[1,2]

See also case GIT4.

### References

1   Kennedy, M. A. (2020). Feline infectious peritonitis: Update on pathogenesis, diagnostics, and treatment. *Veterinary Clinics of North America. Small Animal Practice*, *50*(5), 1001–1011. https://doi.org/10.1016/j.cvsm.2020.05.002

2   Felten, S., & Hartmann, K. (2019). Diagnosis of feline infectious peritonitis: A review of the current literature. *Viruses*, *11*(11), 1068. https://doi.org/10.3390/v11111068

# RESP11 answers

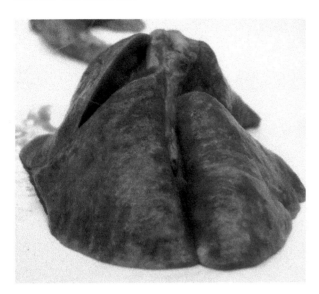

Fig. 4.15

## 1.  Describe any abnormalities

The lungs have failed to collapse and are diffusely mottled dark red to pink with multifocal to coalescing off-white to tan or grey, approximately 1–5 mm foci throughout all lobes.

> Note: These lungs were firmer than normal, something that is not possible to appreciate from the image alone but it is an important feature.

## 2.  Provide a diagnosis

Severe, diffuse, interstitial pneumonia.

## 3.  List some potential causes for this diagnosis

Interstitial pneumonia in cats may be caused by a wide variety of conditions including infectious and non-infectious causes.[1] Some cases are considered idiopathic due to the lack of an identifiable cause. Infectious causes may include virulent calicivirus, pulmonary cowpox, feline herpes virus, pulmonary mycobacteriosis (due to haematogenous spread from lesions elsewhere) and toxoplasmosis.[2,3,4] Non-infectious causes may include diffuse alveolar damage due to sepsis (or systemic inflammation) or inhalation of toxic gases e.g. smoke inhalation or exposure to high concentrations of oxygen (>85%), clinically designated acute respiratory distress syndrome, although termed diffuse alveolar damage histologically.[5] Idiopathic pulmonary

fibrosis is also recognised in cats, but the lesions are often more nodular.

Note: You may have given a diagnosis of neoplasia for part 2. While this was a case of interstitial pneumonia, neoplasia is a reasonable differential. Whether primary or secondary, neoplasms in feline lungs may present as single masses, multifocal masses or as a diffuse pattern.[6,7,8] Primary pulmonary neoplasia in the cat is most likely to be a carcinoma or adenocarcinoma.[7]

## References

1  Caswell, J. L., & Williams, K. J. (2016). Respiratory system. In M. G. Maxie (Ed.), *Jubb, Kennedy and Palmer's pathology of domestic animals* (6th ed), Vol. 2. Elsevier. https://doi.org/10.1016/B978-0-7020-5318-4.00011-5

2  Hofmann-Lehmann, R., Hosie, M. J., Hartmann, K., Egberink H., Truyen, U., Tasker, S., Belák, S., Boucraut-Baralon, C., Frymus, T., Lloret, A., Marsilio, F., Pennisi, M. G., Addie, D. D., Lutz, H., Thiry, E., Radford, A. D., & Möstl, K. (2022, April 29). Calicivirus infection in cats. *Viruses, 14*(5), 937. https://doi.org/10.3390/v14050937

3  McInerney, J., Papasouliotis, K., Simpson, K., English, K., Cook, S., Milne, E., & Gunn-Moore, D. A. (2016). Pulmonary cowpox in cats: Five cases. *Journal of Feline Medicine and Surgery, 18*(6), 518–525. https://doi.org/10.1177/1098612X15583344

4  Gunn-Moore, D. A. (2014, August). Feline mycobacterial infections. *Veterinary Journal, 201*(2), 230–238. https://doi.org/10.1016/j.tvjl.2014.02.014

5  Balakrishnan, A., Drobatz, K. J., & Silverstein, D. C. (2017). Retrospective evaluation of the prevalence, risk factors, management, outcome, and necropsy findings of acute lung injury and acute respiratory distress syndrome in dogs and cats: 29 cases (2011–2013). *Journal of Veterinary Emergency and Critical Care, 27*(6), 662–673. https://doi.org/10.1111/vec.12648

6  Barr, F., Gruffydd-Jones, T. J., Brown, P. J., & Gibbs, C. (1987). Primary lung tumours in the cat. *Journal of Small Animal Practice, 28*(12), 1115–1125. https://doi.org/10.1111/j.1748-5827.1987.tb01336.x

7  Hahn, K. A., & McEntee, M. F. (1997). Primary lung tumor in cats: 86 cases (1979–1994). *Journal of the American Veterinary Medical Association, 211*(10), 1257–1260.

8  Geyer, N. E., Reichle, J. K., Valdés-Martínez, A., Williams, J., Goggin, J. M., Leach, L., Hanson, J., Hill, S., & Axam, T. (2010) Radiographic appearance of confirmed pulmonary lymphoma in cats and dogs. *Veterinary Radiology and Ultrasound, 51*(4), 386–390. https://doi.org/10.1111/j.1740-8261.2010.01683.x

# Hepatic cases

**5**

# HEP1

## Topics

- **Lesion recognition**
- **Generation of pathological differential diagnoses lists**
- **Pathogenesis**
- **Practical technique**

## History

Fig. 5.1 is an image from the abdominal cavity of a 6Y old, female neutered Standard Poodle. The photograph was taken at necropsy.

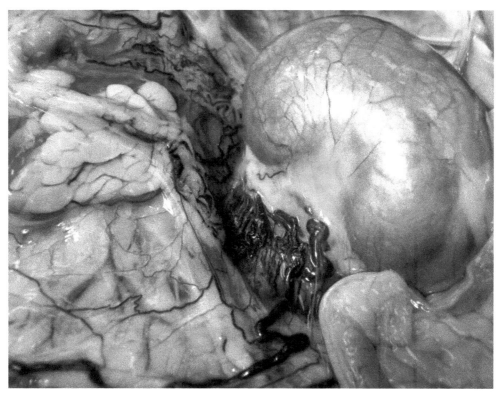

Fig. 5.1

## Questions

1. Describe any abnormalities.
2. Provide a diagnosis.
3. Which organ would you be most interested in examining and what would be your approach to that organ in terms of assessing its disease status? Justify your answer.

# HEP2

## Topics

Lesion recognition

Integration of pathological findings with clinical aspects

Pathogenesis

## History

This liver (Fig. 5.2) originated from a 12Y old, intact female crossbreed dog with a brief history of inappetance, vomiting, lethargy, icterus and abdominal swelling. Necropsy confirmed generalised icterus, moderate ascites and areas of ecchymotic haemorrhage in the intestinal mucosa and peritoneal surface. However, the most severe lesions were in the liver.

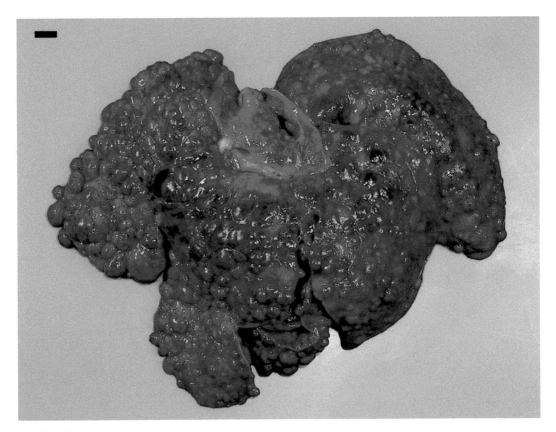

Fig. 5.2  Bar = 1 cm.

## Questions

1. Describe any abnormalities.
2. Provide a diagnosis.
3. Explain how you could integrate the main pathological findings.

# HEP3

## Topic

**Common artefacts and pitfalls**

## History

Fig. 5.3 depicts some gross findings in a 5Y old male Beagle that had been put to sleep due to epilepsy that was refractory to treatment.

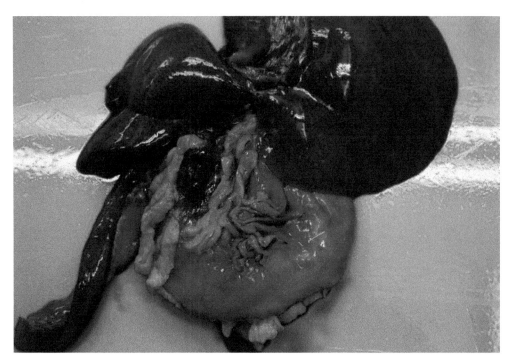

Fig. 5.3

## Questions

1. Describe any abnormalities.
2. Provide a diagnosis.
3. How does this change differ from pseudomelanosis?

# HEP4

## Topic

**Lesion recognition**

## History

This lesion was submitted as a surgical biopsy from a middle-aged Cocker Spaniel. It was detected during abdominal ultrasound examination for an unrelated disorder.

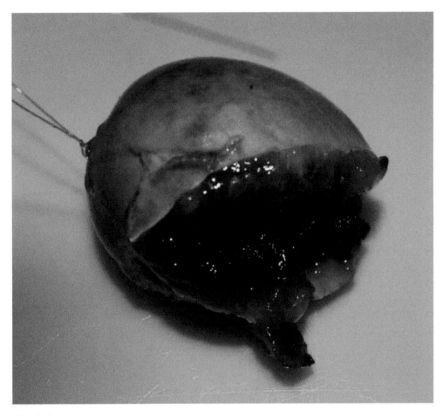

Fig. 5.4

## Questions

1. Describe any abnormalities.
2. Provide a diagnosis.
3. What is the clinical significance of this lesion?

# HEP5

## Topics

Lesion recognition

Generation of pathological differential diagnoses lists

Pathogenesis

## History

Fig. 5.5 shows the main gross lesion discovered during necropsy of a 10Y old, female Chihuahua.

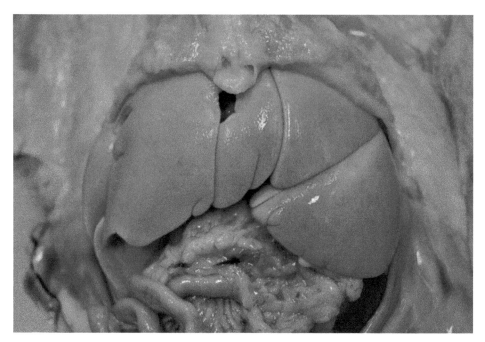

Fig. 5.5

## Questions

1. Describe any abnormalities.
2. Provide a diagnosis.
3. What are the main *pathological* causes of this lesion in the dog (you should be able to list at least **THREE**)?

# HEP6

## Topics

**Lesion recognition**

**Integration of pathological findings with clinical aspects**

## History

Necropsy finding in 11Y old, male Labrador crossbreed euthanised due to anorexia, abdominal discomfort, anaemia and profound lethargy.

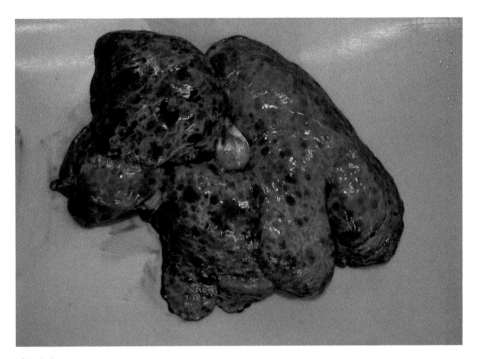

Fig. 5.6

## Questions

1. Describe any abnormalities.
2. Provide a diagnosis.
3. Name **ONE** additional haematological abnormality that might arise in a blood smear.

# HEP7

## Topics

Lesion recognition

Generation of pathological differential diagnoses lists

Health and safety

## History

A 3Y old, male neutered Cocker Spaniel died during early clinical intervention for sudden onset lethargy, vomiting and collapse. The most significant necropsy finding is illustrated in Fig. 5.7. The liver was also friable.

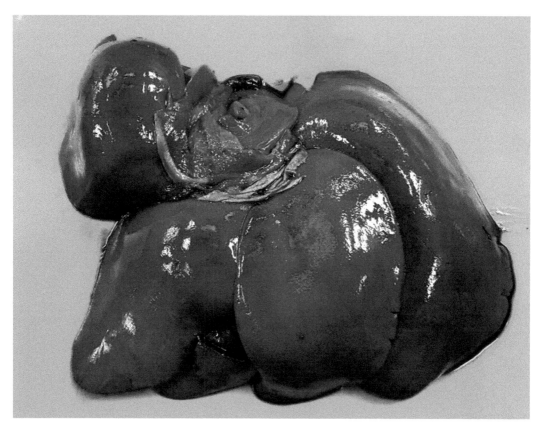

Fig. 5.7

## Questions

1. Describe any abnormalities.
2. Provide a diagnosis.
3. Provide some differential diagnoses for this lesion.

# HEP8

## Topics

Lesion recognition

Generation of pathological differential diagnoses lists

Pathogenesis

## History

An 8Y old, terrier dog presented clinically with ascites. Haematology and a complete blood count were normal and renal function parameters were within normal limits. Biochemistry indicated that alkaline phosphatase (ALP) and aspartate aminotransferase (AST) levels were moderately elevated. The dog died during hospitalisation and a necropsy was undertaken. Fig. 5.8 depicts one of the main necropsy findings. Ascites was also confirmed, along with mild hydropericardium and hydrothorax. The kidneys were grossly normal.

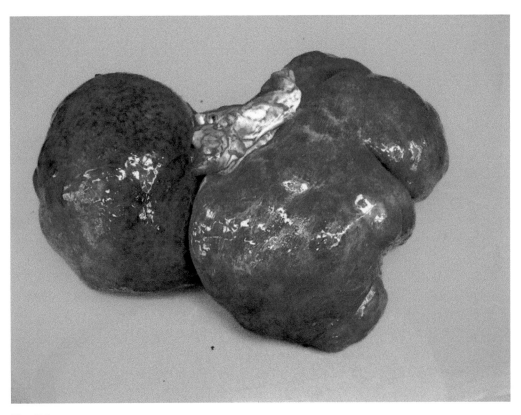

Fig. 5.8

## Questions

1. Describe any abnormalities.
2. Provide a diagnosis.
3. Outline some possible underlying conditions to start ruling out at necropsy and summarise how this lesion develops.

# HEP9

## Topics

Lesion recognition

Health and safety

## History

An 8-week-old, male Labradoodle recently purchased from a farm developed sudden onset malaise, with vomiting and anorexia. The puppy deteriorated despite symptomatic treatment and there was concern regarding leptospirosis. At necropsy, the body was icteric. The other main gross findings are illustrated in Figs 5.9 and 5.10.

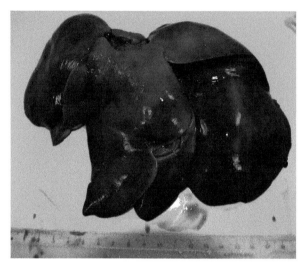

Fig. 5.9

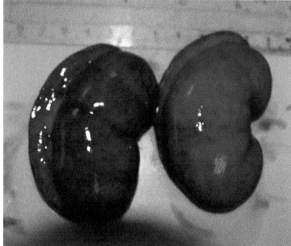

Fig. 5.10

## Questions

1. Describe any abnormalities.
2. Provide a diagnosis.
3. Given the clinical history:
   a) What extra precautions would you advise when undertaking this necropsy?
   b) What samples would you retain for further testing?

# HEP10

## Topics

**Lesion recognition**

**Pathogenesis**

## History and signalment

A 9Y old, female neutered Miniature Schnauzer with a history of diabetes mellitus is submitted for necropsy following a short period of anorexia, vomiting, abdominal pain and a ketoacidotic crisis. At necropsy, the main finding was in the thoracic cavity (Fig. 5.11). There was a moderate serosanguineous peritoneal effusion and numerous peritoneal adhesions. The major changes noted during the necropsy were in the pancreas, peripancreatic fat and liver (as shown below in Figs 5.11 and 5.12).

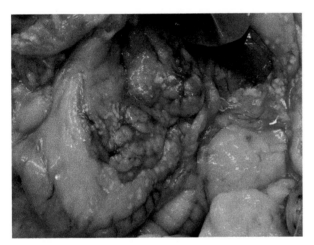

Fig. 5.11

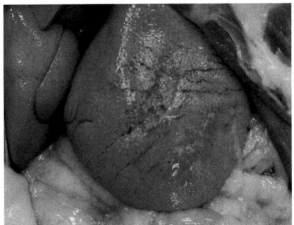

Fig. 5.12

## Questions

1. Describe any abnormalities.
2. Provide a diagnosis.
3. Briefly outline the pathogenesis and suggest where else in the body you may see lesions in dogs with this condition.

# HEP1 answers

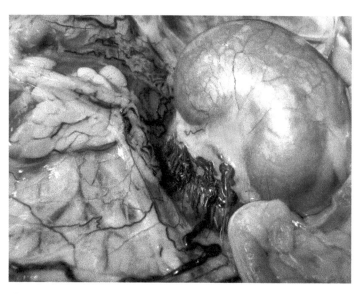

Fig. 5.1

## 1. Describe any abnormalities

Medial to the kidney there are multiple dark red, tortuous blood vessels that cluster close to the hilus but extend randomly into the adjacent fat.

## 2. Provide a diagnosis

Multiple extra-hepatic portosystemic shunts – abdominal cavity.

## 3. Which organ would you be most interested in examining and what would be your approach to that organ in terms of assessing its disease status? Justify your answer.

The liver would be of most interest. Portosystemic shunts (PSS) may be congenital or acquired. Acquired shunts are usually multiple and extra-hepatic while congenital shunts are usually solitary, although they may be extra-hepatic or intra-hepatic. Congenital shunts are more likely to be extra-hepatic in small dogs; Yorkshire Terriers are particularly predisposed, as are Maltese Terriers and Pugs.[1] Acquired shunts generally flag portal hypertension and they form as the body's attempt to maintain normal portal pressure. Portal hypertension can be pre-hepatic, hepatic or post-hepatic in origin but is most commonly hepatic, and often the result of chronic liver disease. It is possible for extra-hepatic shunts to arise secondary to intra-hepatic shunts so, in this case, it would still be worth checking for a shunt within the liver, as far as practically possible. Imaging is also, of course, a very helpful clinical tool.

Postmortem assessment of the liver would include weighing the organ and calculating a percentage body weight (normal in the dog ranges from 2.5–3.9%);[2] evaluating colour, texture, consistency (often firmer in chronic hepatitis) and any other pertinent changes; collecting samples into 10% NBF (minimum of three random samples from more than one lobe, plus any distinct lesions); retaining a sample frozen – this would be potentially useful for toxicology or copper analysis, though copper analysis can be performed on fixed tissue.

> **TIP**
> - Remove the liver and gall bladder with the duodenum, pancreas and stomach (see necropsy sampling guidelines).
> - Open the duodenum and gently squeeze the gall gladder to express bile and ensure patency of the bile duct.
> - Separate liver and gall bladder from other organs and empty gall bladder.
> - Weigh the liver.

## References

1 Tobias, K. M., & Rohrbach, B. W. (2003). Association of breed with the diagnosis of congenital portosystemic shunts in dogs: 2,400 cases (1980–2002). *Journal of the American Veterinary Medical Association, 223*(11), 1636–1639. https://doi.org/10.2460/javma.2003.223.1636

2 McDonough, S.P., & Southard, T. (Eds.) (2016). *Necropsy guide for dogs, cats, and small mammals.* Wiley. http://doi.org.10.1002/9781119317005

# HEP2 answers

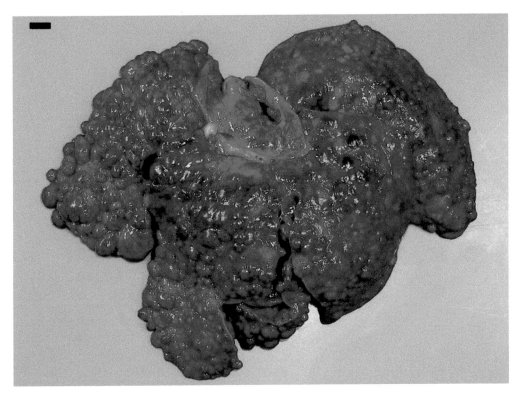

Fig. 5.2 Bar = 1 cm.

## 1.  Describe any abnormalities

The liver is diffusely brick red to tan (normally should be dark 'mahogany' brown). The normal parenchyma is replaced by multifocal to coalescing, raised, shiny, smooth, spherical nodules that range in diameter up to approximately 1.5 cm.

While not appreciable from the image, the parenchyma was much firmer than normal.

## 2.  Provide a diagnosis

This is hepatic cirrhosis (macronodular).

Cirrhosis is an end-stage condition that can be caused by previous infection (e.g. canine adenovirus type 1; *Leptospira* spp.), historical toxin exposure, prolonged therapy with potentially hepatotoxic drugs (e.g. phenobarbital, lomustine, phenytoin), copper toxicosis or chronic interface hepatitis. Definitions vary but the current accepted features are that it is a diffuse process with fibrosis and replacement of normal liver parenchyma by abnormal regenerative nodules.[1] Other features that typically occur include biliary hyperplasia and, by definition, there is also prior injury and loss of hepatocytes.

## 3.  Explain how you could integrate the main pathological findings

The main pathological findings are cirrhosis, icterus, ascites and areas of haemorrhage. Icterus is a clinically and pathologically appreciable manifestation of increased circulating bilirubin, as well as other bile pigments. The main mechanisms are haemolysis (pre-hepatic), hepatocellular injury (hepatic) and obstruction (post-hepatic). Icterus can occur in advanced cases of cirrhosis (due to hepatic insufficiency) but other indicators that may appear before this are ascites and an increased risk of haemorrhage. Ascites is a consequence of hypoproteinaemia and reduced oncotic pressure while haemorrhage may occur due to reduced coagulation factor production by the diseased liver.

### Reference

1  Cullen, J. M. (2009). Summary of the world small animal veterinary association standardisation committee guide to classification of liver disease in dogs and cats. *Veterinary Clinics of North America. Small Animal Practice*, 39(3), 395–418. https://doi.org/10.1016/j.cvsm.2009.02.003

# HEP3 answers

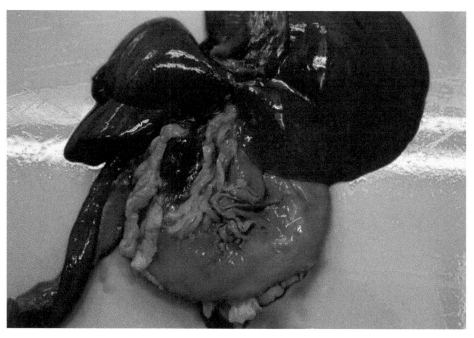

Fig. 5.3

## 1.   Describe any abnormalities

There is focally extensive green and yellow discolouration of the gastric serosa and attached omental fat. There are also multiple, subtle, faintly visible tan lesions throughout the liver, measuring up to ~5 mm diameter.

## 2.   Provide a diagnosis

The green/yellow discolouration is bile imbibition, a common postmortem change. It is another artefact. Bile imbibition results from leakage of bile pigment from the gall bladder to the adjacent soft tissues. The tan foci in the liver may be small areas of fatty change or foci of chronic inflammation; they are likely to be incidental.

## 3.   How does this change differ from pseudomelanosis?

Bile imbibition is the leaching of bile pigment from the gall bladder and bile duct onto the surface of adjacent organs. It results in yellow green discolouration of the affected tissues. Pseudomelanosis, in contrast, manifests as green/black discolouration and is more likely to occur in the intestinal tract. Intestinal bacteria convert iron (originating from autolysed haemoglobin) to iron sulphide. The discolouration can extend to organs adjacent to the gastrointestinal tract, e.g. the kidney. One practical point to make is that it is better to avoid sampling of affected areas as they are likely to be a little more autolysed than non-discoloured tissues.

# HEP4 answers

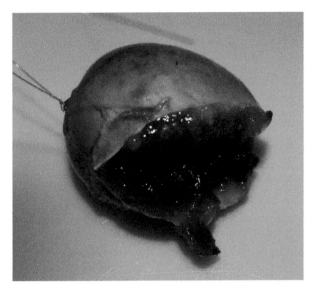

Fig. 5.4

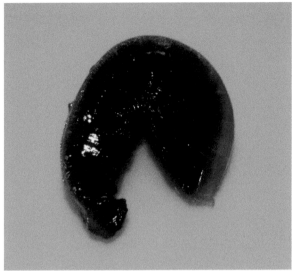

Fig. 5.4a Transverse section through a gall bladder mucocoele, canine.

## 1.    Describe any abnormalities

This specimen contains no recognisable architecture. It comprises part of a rounded (ovoid or spherical), soft, bulging, dark green mass that is circumscribed by a thin grey, opaque membrane.

## 2.    Provide a diagnosis

This lesion is **NOT** a burst, over-ripe kiwi fruit or green-gage. It is a gall bladder mucocoele and is characterised by dilation of the gall bladder by mucoid material. The mucosa is hyperplastic and forms fronds surrounding cystic spaces filled with mucus. Fig. 5.4a is a transverse section across a gall bladder mucocoele, illustrating the semi-solid nature of the excess mucus secretion.

## 3.    What is the clinical significance of this lesion?

In severe cases, the wall of the gall bladder can become necrotic so there is the risk of rupture and bile peritonitis. However, many cases develop slowly so may not have any clinical signs and are detected as an apparently incidental finding (i.e. clinically irrelevant), at least at that stage.[1] Cocker Spaniels are predisposed but Miniature Schnauzers

and Shetland Sheepdogs are also vulnerable to this disorder.[2,3,4] The cause of this lesion has not been established, but animals with endocrinopathies are reported to have an increased risk of developing this condition. Other speculated causes have included progestin therapy, cholecystitis, biliary stasis and increased bile viscosity or 'sludging' but the cause remains unproven.[4]

## References

1   Ettinger, S. J., Feldman, E. C., & Côté, E. (2017). *Textbook of veterinary internal medicine.* Saunders.

2   Norwich, A. (2011). Gallbladder mucocele in a 12-year-old cocker spaniel. *Canadian Veterinary Journal, 52*(3), 319–321.

3   Aguirre, A. L., Center, S. A., Randolph, J. F., Yeager, A. E., Keegan, A. M., Harvey, H. J., & Erb, H. N. (2007). Gallbladder disease in Shetland sheepdogs: 38 cases (1995–2005). *Journal of the American Veterinary Medical Association, 231*(1), 79–88. https://doi.org/10.2460/javma.231.1.79

4   Smalle, T. M., Cahalane, A. K., & Köster, L. S. (2015). Gallbladder mucocoele: A review. *Journal of the South African Veterinary Association, 86*(1), 1318. https://doi.org/10.4102/jsava.v86i1.1318

# HEP5 answers

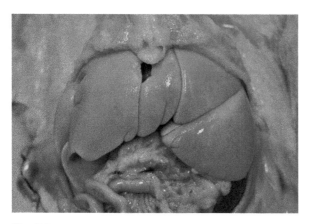

Fig. 5.5

## 1. Describe any abnormalities

The liver is diffusely pale tan/fawn and markedly enlarged, with rounded borders. (It also likely had a greasy texture though this is not always easy to distinguish from an image alone).

## 2. Provide a diagnosis

Severe, diffuse hepatic fatty change (or hepatic lipidosis).

## 3. What are the main *pathological* causes of this lesion in the dog (you should be able to list at least **THREE**)?

The most common cause of diffuse hepatic fatty change (lipidosis) is anorexia and this, of course, can occur for lots of reasons.[1] Fatty change in the liver is also often associated with endocrine disease (diabetes mellitus, hypothyroidism, hyperadrenocorticism and pancreatitis[2]). It may be idiopathic (i.e. primary or at least of unknown cause) – examples include primary idiopathic hyperlipidaemia in the Schnauzer and hepatic lipidosis in toy breeds of dog.[1,2] The idiopathic form is much more common in the cat, however.[1]

In this condition, there is excessive accumulation of lipid within hepatocytes, leading to cell swelling and cytoplasmic vacuolation. Mechanistically, the causes of fatty change can be divided into one of three main categories.

- Increased mobilisation of peripheral fat to the liver, in the form of free fatty acids. This is more likely to happen if the dog has stopped eating for some reason (including malnourishment/neglect/ starvation).
- Abnormal lipid metabolism by hepatocytes. Diseased hepatocytes are unable to adequately process and metabolise various lipid components (fatty acids, triglycerides, apoproteins).

- Diminished release of lipoproteins. Apoproteins are responsible for transporting fatty acids out of the liver once they have been converted to triglycerides. The triglycerides and apoproteins combine to form lipoproteins which are then eliminated from the liver. Anything that inhibits this pathway may lead to lipidosis (e.g. starvation may deprive the animal of sufficient apoproteins).[1]

Basically, fatty change in the liver is an indicator of an energy imbalance. Note that hepatic fatty change may be a consequence of non-pathological processes (physiological) or high fat diet, though these reasons are less likely in the dog and cat.

Fig. 5.5a is another case of hepatic fatty change but it illustrates an additional feature, which is that the severely affected fatty liver is often very friable, which may predispose it to fracturing and, ultimately, haemorrhage, which can be sufficiently significant to lead to death.

> Note there are also some yellow foci of necrosis that are not directly related to the lipidosis – also see HEP10.

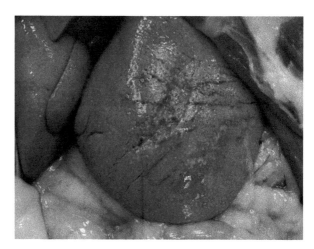

Fig. 5.5a **Canine liver with severe fatty change.**

## References

1 Cullen, J. M., & Stalker, M. J. (2016). Liver and biliary system. M. G. Maxie (Ed.), *Jubb, Kennedy and Palmer's pathology of domestic animals* (6th ed), Vol. 2 (pp. 275–277). Elsevier. https://doi.org/10.1016/B978-0-7020-5318-4.00008-5

2 Xenoulis, P. G., & Steiner, J. M. (2010). Lipid metabolism and hyperlipidemia in dogs. Veterinary Journal, 183(1), 12–21. https://doi.org/10.1016/j.tvjl.2008.10.011

# HEP6 answers

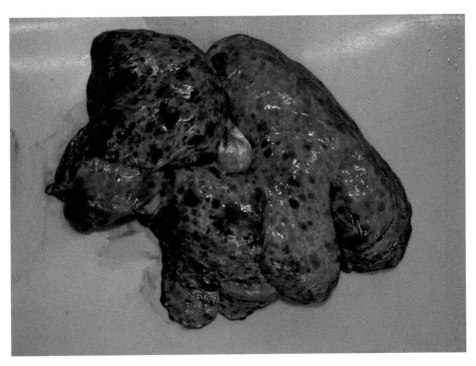

Fig. 5.6

## 1. Describe any abnormalities

Disseminated throughout all liver lobes are innumerable, multifocal to coalescing, well-demarcated, dark red/purple, translucent lesions that are mostly flush with the capsular surface. They range from pinpoint to approximately 2 cm diameter. The liver is also diffusely enlarged and orange/tan with rounded borders.

## 2. Provide a diagnosis

Metastatic haemangiosarcoma. The multifocal pattern is consistent with metastasis. The dark red translucency is very characteristic of this malignant tumour of endothelial cell origin. The question does not provide sufficient information to allow definitive diagnosis of organ of origin. It would be important to examine other common primary sites (right atrium of the heart, spleen, possibly kidney and skin) and, if no evidence of any haemangiosarcoma there, then this could well be of hepatic origin, with intra-hepatic metastasis. In such a case, we might expect to see metastases to other organs, particularly the lungs and perhaps the brain.

The concurrent generalised enlargement, orange/tan colour and rounded borders likely reflect fatty change secondary to inappetence and/or due to the effects of the haemangiosarcoma, e.g. anaemia following blood loss.

## 3. Name ONE additional haematological abnormality that might arise in a blood smear

Regenerative anaemia (e.g. reticulocytosis, polychromasia) may arise due to internal haemorrhage associated with this type of neoplasm. Acanthocytes, schistocytes or keratocytes may be seen in conjunction with haemangiosarcoma since circulation of red blood cells through abnormal vasculature leads to cell damage and abnormal shapes.

Acanthocytes: Red blood cells (RBCs) with irregular cytoplasmic projections.
Schistocytes: Fragmented RBCs.
Keratocytes: RBCs with blister-like projections.

# HEP7 answers

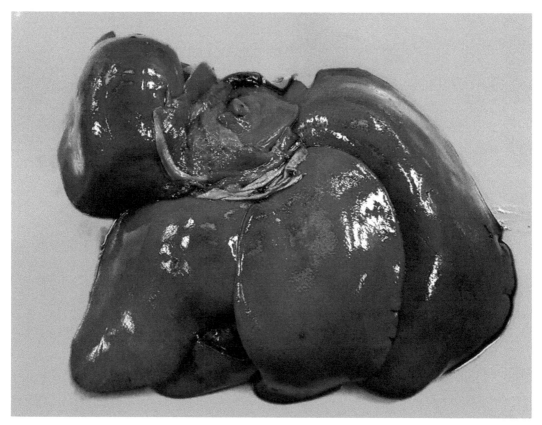

Fig. 5.7

## 1.   Describe any abnormalities

The liver is diffusely pale brown/tan (certainly paler than normal) with slightly rounded borders in some lobes. There is also a subtle red pinpoint speckling of the liver.

## 2.   Provide a diagnosis

Severe diffuse acute hepatocellular necrosis.

A reasonable gross differential is acute necrotising hepatitis so take credit for that too. Differentiating between these two requires histopathology.

> Note: In 'real life' we would be able to assess the consistency of the liver – we obviously cannot do that from this particular image which is why we gave you the extra clue of increased friability. Necrotic livers are generally more friable than normal. This can be evaluated by applying some pressure with the fingers. If the thumb can penetrate the parenchyma with just a little pressure, this indicates increased friability and suggests necrosis. Features that support an acute condition in this case are the lack of any tissue loss or repair processes (such as fibrosis or nodular regeneration). These would likely change the shape of the liver, rendering it more irregular and firmer.

## 3.   Provide some differential diagnoses for this lesion

Differentials should include causes of diffuse acute (necrotising) hepatitis and diffuse acute hepatic necrosis since, to all intents and purposes, these cannot really be distinguished from each other grossly. Histopathology not only helps to separate primary inflammation from primary necrosis, but it also helps to determine the *pattern* of necrosis, key to narrowing down potential causes, though typically not enough to pinpoint exactly. That is where toxicology and culture come in. It is thus important to retain fixed **and** fresh liver, to allow for histopathology and other types of testing.

- Acute hepatitis:
  canine adenovirus type 1 (infectious canine hepatitis)
  *Leptospira* spp.*
  consider herpesvirus in neonates
  *Clostridium piliforme* (Tyzzer's disease). Though this usually presents as multiple white foci, it is still worth ruling out.
- Acute hepatic necrosis:
  drugs, e.g. acetaminophen (paracetamol) at high doses; xylitol (artificial sweetener)

blue green algae (cyanobacteria)

idiosyncratic drug reactions (trimethoprim-sulfonamide, carprofen)

toxic fungi (e.g. *Amanita*, which does occur in the UK)[1]

aflatoxins (via contamination of dog food)

hypoxia, e.g. due to severe anaemia[†]

*Salmonella* has also been reported as a cause.[2]

Other conditions can make the liver diffusely paler than normal, such as lipidosis, amyloidosis and infiltrative neoplasia, but they are usually accompanied by more pronounced enlargement of the liver with accentuated rounding of lobe margins. Amyloidosis confers a more turgid, waxy consistency, as opposed to increased friability. Nevertheless, histopathology will generally be sufficient to exclude these other considerations.

## Notes

*Main species are: *autumnalis, bratislava, canicola, grippotyphosa, icterohaemorrhagiae, pomona*.

†Which was the cause in this case, a consequence of immune-mediated haemolytic anaemia (IMHA)

Leptospira is potentially zoonotic, so do bear that in mind when handling fresh tissues. Consider double gloving and additional personal protective equipment, such as safety goggles and cut resistant gloves.

TIP

This particular case is quite subtle, but it demonstrates how it can sometimes (often) be difficult to appreciate acute hepatocellular necrosis – it can even be mistaken for mild lipidosis. For these reasons, always sample three or four liver lobes to ensure you have portions that are as representative as possible.

Final note: Even histologically, necrotising hepatitis and hepatic necrosis can be difficult to distinguish from each other as inflammation and necrosis are often present in both processes. Unravelling these cases and determining likely cause depends on deciding which came first and this is not always possible.

## References

1   Puschner, B., Rose, H. H., & Filigenzi, M. S. (2007). Diagnosis of *Amanita* toxicosis in a dog with acute hepatic necrosis. *Journal of Veterinary Diagnostic Investigation*, *19*(3), 312–317. https://doi.org/10.1177/104063870701900317

2   Meiring, G. A., Grant, A. J., & Watson, P. J. (2015). Acute hepatic necrosis caused by *Salmonella enterica* serotype I 4,5,12:-:1,2 in a dog. *Journal of Clinical Microbiology*, *53*, 3674–3676. https://doi.org/10.1128/JCM.01256-15

# HEP8 answers

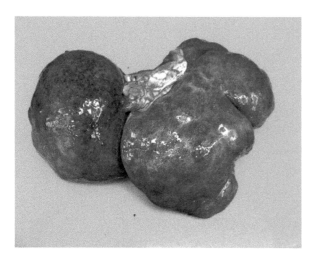

Fig. 5.8

## 1. Describe any abnormalities

The liver is diffusely markedly enlarged and mottled brick red and dark red, with rounded borders and an irregular surface.

## 2. Provide a diagnosis

Severe, diffuse, chronic, passive congestion.

## 3. Outline some possible underlying conditions to start ruling out at necropsy and summarise how this lesion develops

In chronic passive congestion, the hepatic sinusoids, particularly those around central veins, become dilated and engorged with blood. This is usually due to 'damming back' of blood. Normally, blood courses into the liver via the hepatic artery and portal vein (i.e. it enters through the portal tracts); it travels through the sinusoids and exits via the hepatic vein (the central vein). From there it enters the caudal vena cava and flows to the right atrium of the heart. Anything along that route that obstructs or slows outflow of blood from the liver has the potential to cause damming back and centrilobular sinusoidal dilation. If sufficiently severe, this could theoretically involve midzonal and periportal sinusoids but, in practice, it is centrilobular areas that tend to be very congested. This confers a zonal

red appearance grossly. At the same time, there may be slowing of blood flow into the liver with fatty change in the periportal hepatocytes, fibrosis and increased nodularity. Conditions to consider are right heart failure, left heart failure leading to right heart failure, and/or impeded blood flow through the hepatic veins and caudal vena cava. The zonality leads to a gross appearance on cut section that resembles a nutmeg, hence the colloquial term for this condition – 'nutmeg liver' (Figs 5.8a and b).

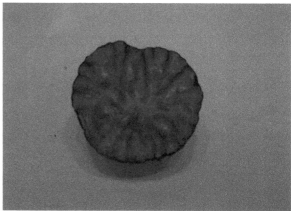

Fig. 5.8a **Cross section of a nutmeg.**

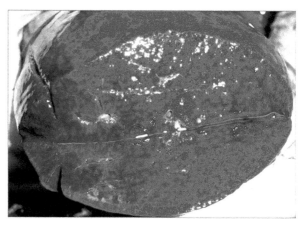

Fig. 5.8b **Hepatic chronic passive congestion ('nutmeg liver') in a dog with dilated cardiomyopathy.**

# HEP9 answers

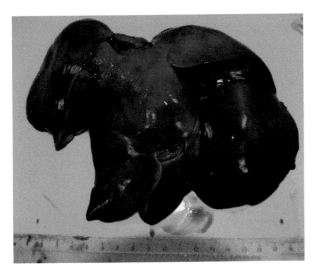

Fig. 5.9

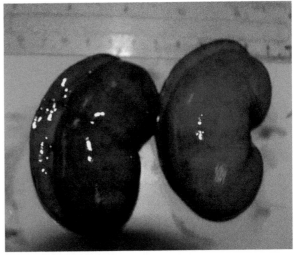

Fig. 5.10

## 1.  Describe any abnormalities

The liver is flaccid and mottled orange to red-brown with ill-defined, darker red areas. The kidneys are diffusely tan with marked, red to purple mottling of the cortical surfaces. There is also mild petechial haemorrhage on the cortical surface.

## 2.  Provide a diagnosis

a. Severe diffuse acute hepatic necrosis.
b. Severe diffuse acute bilateral nephropathy with petechial haemorrhage (likely acute tubular necrosis given the diffuse pallor).

These changes are suggestive of leptospirosis and further testing was advised (see below for information on further testing).

## 3.  Given the clinical history

a)  What extra precautions would you advise when undertaking this necropsy?

When considering undertaking a necropsy on a potentially zoonotic case you should consider all in-contact staff and any underlying health concerns (e.g. are any staff potentially immunosuppressed, pregnant etc.), as well as your ability to manage the risk of infection e.g. containment of infection and disinfection of the area afterwards; disposable protective personal equipment (including eye glasses), double gloving and anti-cut gloves are all advised. If you are concerned that the infection risk cannot be contained, then consider sending to a laboratory with appropriate facilities.

b)  What samples would you retain for further testing?

Formalin-fixed samples of liver and kidney for histology and possible special staining with Warthin-Starry for *Leptospira* spp. or, preferably, more specific tests such as immunohistochemistry. In addition, retain fresh samples of liver and kidney which can be submitted for PCR testing if required.

# HEP10 answers

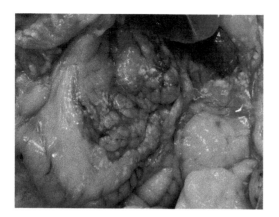

Fig. 5.11

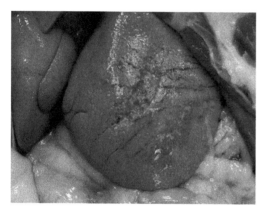

Fig. 5.12

### 1. Describe any abnormalities

Pancreas – The pancreas is irregular with multifocal to coalescing, off-white, 2–3 mm foci, which extend into the peripancreatic fat and are accompanied by red mottling (similar lesions were found in the mesentery, omentum and the perirenal fat – see Fig. 5.12a below).

Liver – The liver is diffusely pale tan with a prominent lobular pattern, bright yellow, depressed foci and mild red mottling. Multiple linear fissures indicate a friable texture.

### 2. Provide a diagnosis

a. Acute pancreatic and peripancreatic fat necrosis (otherwise known as acute necrotising pancreatitis).
b. Hepatic lipidosis and necrosis.

Note: Liver necrosis can occur secondary to pancreatic necrosis – the friable texture in this case was not associated with haemorrhage but increased friability of the liver can lead to fracturing and significant haemorrhage.

### 3. Briefly outline the pathogenesis and suggest where else in the body you may see lesions in dogs with this condition

Release of lipolytic enzymes from the pancreas, such as trypsin and lipase, leads to pancreatic necrosis and peripancreatic fat necrosis. There is often fibrinous inflammation and haemorrhage around the pancreas, as well as chalky white lesions on the pancreas and peripancreatic fat. The inflamed pancreas releases cytokines and inflammatory mediators that result in systemic effects so that the fat necrosis can occur in other parts of the body distant to the pancreas. Animals may develop foci of necrotising panniculitis (and see case CVS8 for a more unusual example).

Note: The colour of the pancreas at time of necropsy can range considerably and still be within normal limits (e.g. white, red, grey, pale yellow, lilac, pink, etc). The pancreas is also prone to deceptive colour changes due to autolysis (see Fig. 5.12b below). However, discrete white lesions such as those in Fig. 5.11 are always abnormal and pancreatic necrosis should always be considered, especially if they encroach on the peripancreatic fat and have a 'chalky' consistency.

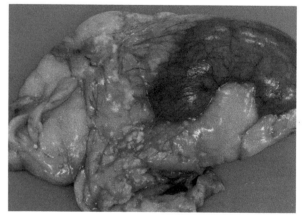

Fig. 5.12a **Acute fat necrosis in the perirenal fat.**

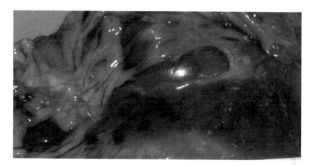

Fig. 5.12b **Autolysed canine pancreas with light to dark red mottling of the parenchyma.**

# Urinary cases

# 6

# URIN1

## Topics

**Lesion recognition**

**Generation of pathological differential diagnoses lists**

**Practical technique**

## History

These kidneys are from a 9Y old, female neutered domestic shorthair cat with a history of intermittent haematuria, dysuria and stranguria.

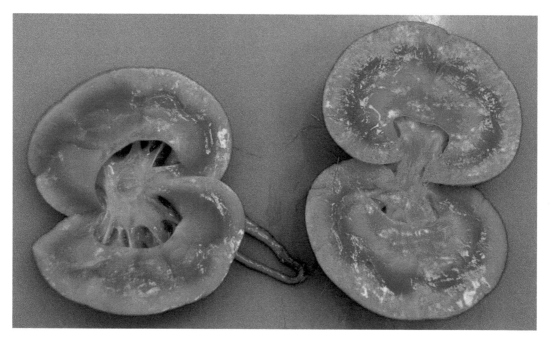

Fig. 6.1

## Questions

1. Describe any abnormalities.
2. Provide a diagnosis.
3. What is the most likely cause and its probable location?

# URIN2

## Topic

**Lesion recognition**

## History

The organ below is from a 14Y old, female Siamese cat with a 2 week history of dysuria and haematuria.

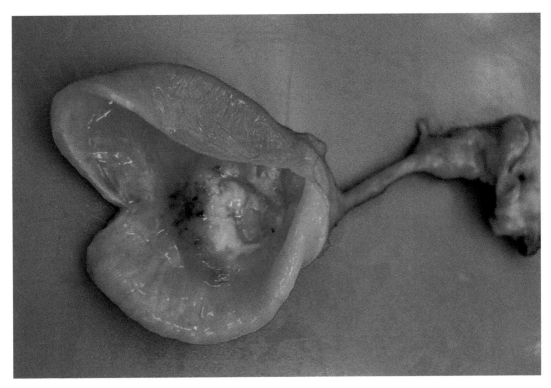

Fig. 6.2

## Questions

1. Describe any abnormalities.
2. Provide a diagnosis.
3. The diagnosis in this particular case was, unexpectedly, a leiomyosarcoma. Define this term.

# URIN3

## Topics

Lesion recognition

Generation of pathological differential diagnoses lists

Pathogenesis

Integration of pathological findings with clinical aspects

## History

A 12Y old, female neutered domestic shorthair cat was euthanised following a period of weight loss, anorexia and dyspnoea. The main necropsy findings were pulmonary oedema, a moderate, low-protein, serosanguineous effusion in the pleural space and peritoneal cavity, and moderate bilateral enlargement of the parathyroid glands. The image in Fig. 6.3 is of one of the kidneys but both kidneys were grossly very similar.

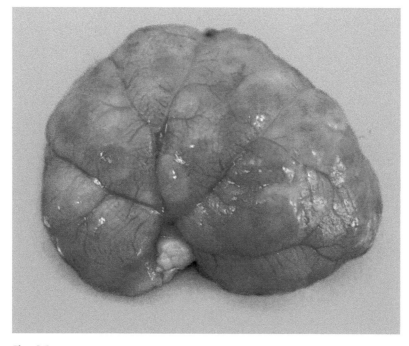

Fig. 6.3

## Questions

1. Describe any abnormalities.
2. Provide a diagnosis.
3. In this case histopathology confirmed lymphoma in the liver, heart and diaphragm. Outline the likely pathogenesis of the cavitary effusions and parathyroid gland enlargement.

# URIN4

## Topics

Practical technique

Lesion recognition

## History

The kidney in Fig. 6.4 was removed from a 10Y old, male neutered Springer Spaniel with a history of haematuria. The other kidney was grossly normal.

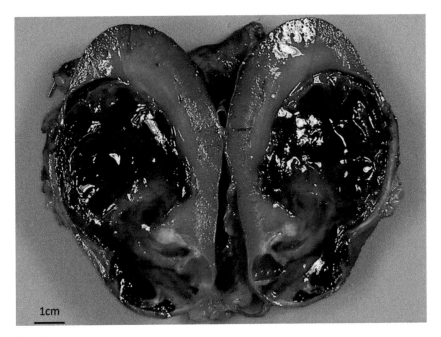

Fig. 6.4

## Questions

1. Describe any abnormalities.
2. Provide a diagnosis.
3. Describe how you would sample and submit this specimen for further testing. Which tests would you consider?

# URIN5

## Topics

**Lesion recognition**

**Generation of pathological differential diagnoses lists**

**Health and safety**

**Pathogenesis**

## History

The kidneys in Fig. 6.5 were collected during the necropsy of a 7Y old, male German Shepherd Dog.

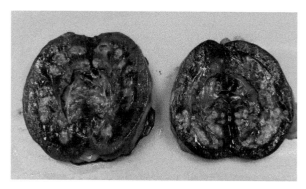

Fig. 6.5

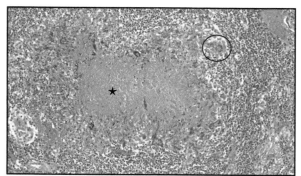

Fig. 6.6

## Questions

1. Describe any abnormalities in Fig. 6.5.
2. Provide a diagnosis.
3. Fig. 6.6 is a histopathological image of one of the lesions. The image does not contain any normal renal architecture. Identify the lesion, justify your reasoning and explain why there might be a health and safety concern with this case.

# URIN6

## Topics

Practical technique

Lesion recognition

Approach to difficult cases

## History

Fig. 6.7 illustrates tissues from a 9-month-old, female Labrador mixed-breed dog. The bitch was euthanised due to a combination of persistent urinary incontinence and behavioural issues.

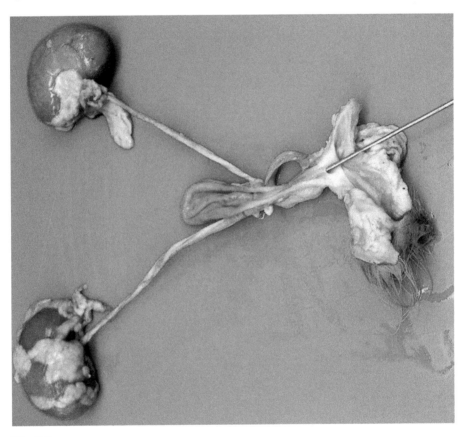

Fig. 6.7

## Questions

1. Describe any abnormalities. HINT: Look at the probe.
2. Provide a diagnosis.
3. Identify the relevant anatomic structures then compare your answer with Fig. 6.7a (labelled in the Answer section).

# URIN7

## Topics

> Lesion recognition

> Practical technique

> Pathogenesis

> Integration of pathological findings with clinical aspects

## History

A male, 7Y old, neutered Pomeranian died and was subsequently presented for necropsy following a 1 week period of anorexia, vomiting and lethargy. Immediately prior to this, it had been treated symptomatically for an unspecified forelimb lameness using a broad-spectrum antimicrobial in conjunction with an oral non-steroidal anti-inflammatory drug (NSAID).

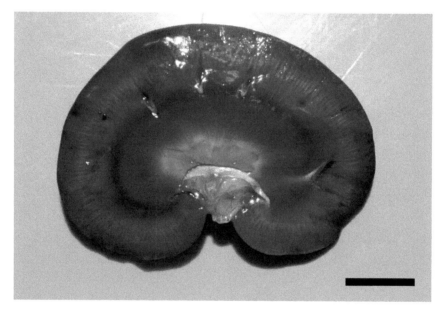

Fig. 6.8 Bar = 1 cm.

## Questions

1. Describe any abnormalities.
2. Provide a diagnosis.
3. Link this lesion to the clinical history and briefly outline the pathogenesis.

# URIN8

## Topics

Lesion recognition

Generation of pathological differential diagnoses lists

## History

Fig. 6.9 depicts the main necropsy finding in a 5Y old, female neutered Labrador that had died despite symptomatic treatment for acute renal failure (she had presented with anorexia, lethargy and vomiting).

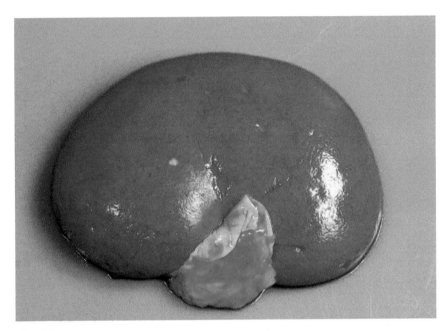

Fig. 6.9

## Questions

1. Describe any abnormalities.
2. Provide a diagnosis.
3. Given the clinical history, what is the most likely cause? List some other potential causes.

# URIN9

## Topics

Lesion recognition

Pathogenesis

## History

Figs 6.10 and 6.11 illustrate the main necropsy finding in a 7Y old, male neutered domestic shorthair cat that had presented collapsed with a history of stranguria and dysuria.

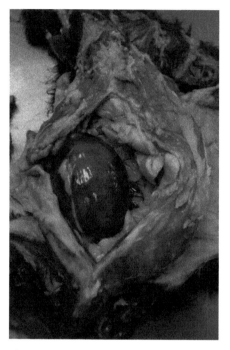

Fig. 6.10

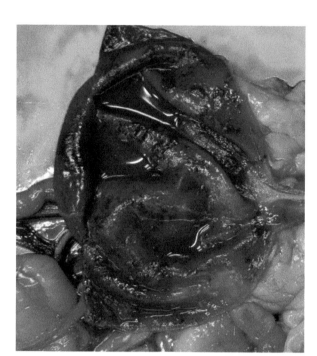

Fig. 6.11

## Questions

1. Describe any abnormalities.
2. Provide a diagnosis.
3. Where should you look next and why?

# URIN10

## Topics

**Lesion recognition**

Pathogenesis

## History

The left kidney was markedly enlarged in a 9Y old male Persian cat. This lesion was palpated when the cat was having a routine dental. The cat was not in renal failure and ultrasound indicated that the right kidney was grossly normal but abdominal palpation elicited some discomfort. The affected kidney was subsequently surgically removed and uroliths were confirmed in the ipsilateral ureter. The cat recovered uneventfully so this is not a necropsy case – but this type of lesion could well be found incidentally at necropsy, although perhaps not as severe.

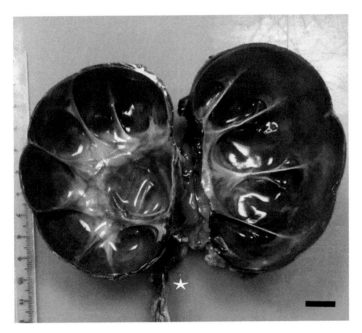

Fig. 6.12  Bar = 1 cm.

## Questions

1. Describe any abnormalities.
2. Provide a diagnosis.
3. What is the underlying pathological process that leads to this lesion?

# URIN11

## Topics

Lesion recognition

Generation of pathological differential diagnoses lists

Integration of pathological findings with clinical aspects

## History

A 10Y old, female neutered terrier mixed-breed dog presented with abdominal pain, haematuria, weight loss and inappetence. Ultrasound detected a mass in the region of the left kidney and a moderate peritoneal effusion that proved to be a transudate on fluid analysis. The owner opted for euthanasia, mainly due to the rapid clinical deterioration of the dog. Fig. 6.13 is an image of both kidneys at the time of necropsy. There were no other gross lesions, apart from mild bilateral degenerative joint disease in the stifles.

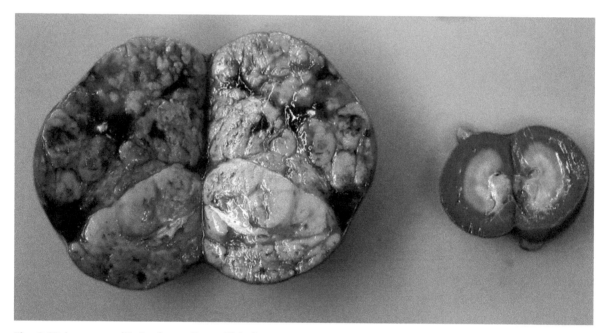

Fig. 6.13 Image credit: Professor Susan Rhind.

## Questions

1. Describe any abnormalities.
2. Provide a diagnosis.
3. How would you link the peritoneal effusion to the renal tumour in this case?

# URIN12

## Topics

**Lesion recognition**

**Pathogenesis**

## History

A 6-month-old, male, crossbreed dog presented with polyuria and polydipsia. The puppy had failed to thrive and was underweight, as well as quite subdued for its age. Further investigations indicated that the puppy had azotaemia, proteinuria, hypoproteinaemia and hypercholesterolaemia. Ultrasound confirmed that both kidneys were misshapen. Eventually, the puppy had to be euthanised due to a diagnosis of severe uraemia and further clinical deterioration. Figs 6.14 and 6.15 depict one of the kidneys at necropsy.

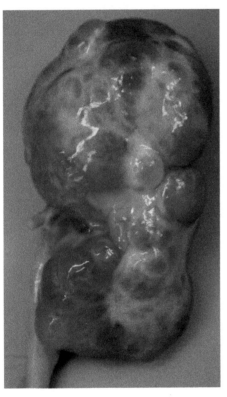

Fig. 6.14

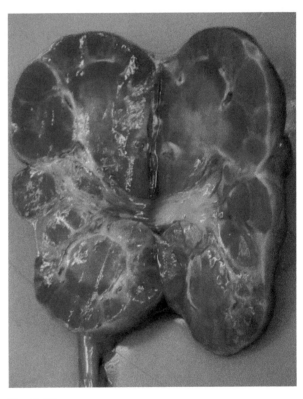

Fig. 6.15

## Questions

1. Describe any abnormalities.
2. Provide a diagnosis.
3. (a) Summarise the pertinent features of this condition.
   (b) Provide at least **FIVE** grossly appreciable necropsy lesions you might expect to find associated with the clinical diagnosis of uraemia.

# URIN1 answers

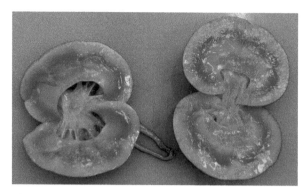

Fig. 6.1

I. Hydronephrosis results in abnormal exposure of renal calyces – the novice may mistake these for areas of fibrosis (scarring). See the arrows in Fig 6.1a which point out these structures – they are normal but not usually visible – loss of the renal parenchyma has exposed them.

Refer to Case URIN10 for an extreme example.

II. Always longitudinally section the kidneys while still in the body cavity. If there is hydronephrosis, this will make it much easier for you to follow the ureter from the kidney to check for an obstruction.

## 1.    Describe any abnormalities

The renal pelvis of the kidney on the left is mildly dilated, exposing the renal calyces. The kidney on the right is grossly normal.

## 2.    Provide a diagnosis

Mild unilateral hydronephrosis.

## 3.    What is the most likely cause and its probable location?

This is due to obstruction of urine outflow. Possible specific causes include urinary calculi (uroliths), neoplasia and iatrogenic (e.g. erroneous clamping of the ureter during neutering). Since the lesion is unilateral, the blockage is most likely in the ipsilateral ureter. Bilateral hydronephrosis may be due to blockage of both ureters or, more likely, blockage in the urinary bladder or urethra.

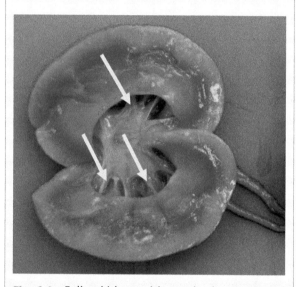

Fig. 6.1a Feline kidney with renal calyces exposed (arrows).

# URIN2 answers

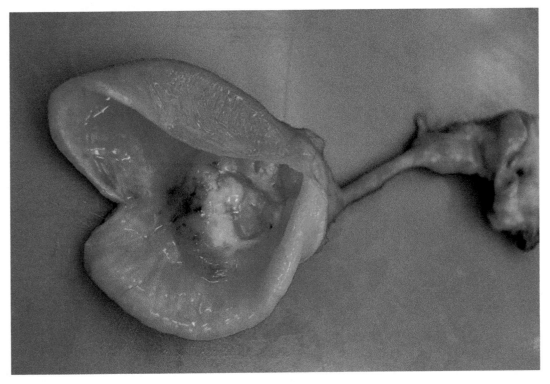

Fig. 6.2

### 1.    Describe any abnormalities

There is focally extensive effacement of the urinary bladder mucosa, mainly in the trigone area, by a well-defined, yellow, raised mass measuring approximately 2 cm diameter. The superimposed red area is consistent with haemorrhage.

### 2.    Provide a diagnosis

'Playing the odds', urothelial (transitional) cell carcinoma is most likely given the age of the cat, location of the tumour and clinical history of haemorrhage. The prognosis is generally poor due to the infiltrative nature of this carcinoma. It tends to invade along the lumen of the urethra and ureters. It can also metastasise, usually to lymph nodes and lungs, but other organs may be involved, including bone.

### 3.    The diagnosis in this particular case was, unexpectedly, a leiomyosarcoma. Define this term.

Leiomyosarcoma is a malignant mesenchymal tumour of smooth muscle origin. It was unexpected in this case since it is much less common. Such tumours are generally locally infiltrative, but they rarely metastasise. The benign equivalent, the leiomyoma, is more common in the genital tract, and then usually in older female dogs.

# URIN3 answers

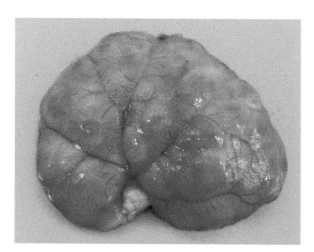

Fig. 6.3

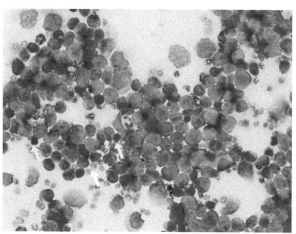

Fig. 6.3a Cytological smear from the lymph node in a different case of feline lymphoma. There is a predominance of large, atypical lymphocytes arranged in sheets with a light background of red blood cells (white arrow), small lymphocytes (yellow arrows) and a neutrophil (red arrow).

## 1.  Describe any abnormalities

The cortical surface is very irregular due to the formation of multifocal to coalescing, smooth, raised, rather ill-defined, pale tan to yellow nodules that range in diameter up to approximately 1 cm.

## 2.  Provide a diagnosis

The most likely differential is lymphoma (confirmed in this case with histopathology) but a reasonable differential would be granulomatous nephritis secondary to feline infectious peritonitis or other round cell neoplasia (mast cell tumour, histiocytic neoplasia). A suspicion of lymphoma could be confirmed using impression smears at time of necropsy, although autolysis can sometimes obscure cell morphology in cytological smears (Fig. 6.3a is a good example of a cytological smear from a case of lymphoma).

## 3.  In this case histopathology confirmed lymphoma in the liver, heart and diaphragm. Outline the likely pathogenesis of the cavitary effusions and parathyroid gland enlargement.

Serosanguineous effusions and pulmonary oedema indicate fluid imbalance which may be a consequence of:

a. increased hydrostatic pressure
b. increased vascular permeability
c. decreased intravascular osmotic pressure
d. reduced lymphatic drainage.

The effusions in this case may have been due to a combination of increased hydrostatic pressure and decreased intravascular osmotic pressure. Lymphoma in the heart may have adversely affected cardiac function, leading to increased hydrostatic pressure. However, it is more likely that renal and hepatic failure combined to reduce intravascular osmotic pressure through protein-losing nephropathy and decreased albumin production by the liver. Neoplastic processes can also limit lymphatic drainage though this is more likely with carcinomas.

The enlarged parathyroid glands support bilateral parathyroid gland hyperplasia secondary to renal failure. If the glomerular filtration rate is affected this can lead to retention of phosphorus and reduced circulating calcium. Chronic renal disease also impairs vitamin D production which adversely impacts on absorption of calcium from the intestine. Either way, the resultant hypocalcaemia triggers increased parathyroid hormone secretion which stimulates hyperplasia of both parathyroid glands. The aim of this is to increase parathyroid hormone levels, in turn facilitating increased resorption of calcium from the bones and re-balancing circulating calcium levels.

# URIN4 answers

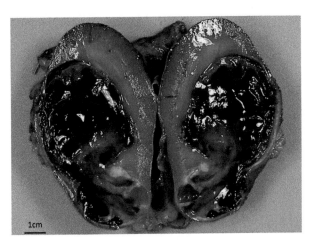

Fig. 6.4

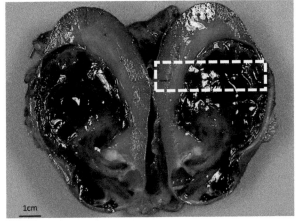

Fig. 6.4a

## 1.  Describe any abnormalities

More than 80% of the renal parenchyma, including the renal papilla, medulla and cortex, is replaced by a well-demarcated, bi-lobed, dark red, gelatinous mass that measures approximately 8 × 4 cm at its widest dimensions.

## 2.  Provide a diagnosis

This is renal haemangiosarcoma. However, based on gross morphology alone other differentials include a haematoma and, much less likely, a haemangioma or vascular anomaly, such as a vascular hamartoma. Despite the very haemorrhagic appearance, urothelial carcinoma probably should not be excluded without histopathological evaluation, although the gross appearance is really not suggestive of that.

## 3.  Describe how you would sample and submit this specimen for further testing. Which tests would you consider?

Half of this kidney could be submitted in 10% neutral buffered formalin (NBF) for histopathology, preferably sliced into thin slabs of appropriate dimensions for optimum fixation. As with other larger samples, complete fixation before packing and sending will allow submission in a smaller volume of NBF. If choosing to send only a representative portion, ensure submission of at least one slice (preferably two or three; see Fig. 6.4a for suggested sampling approach) that includes margin with normal tissue. Submitting only the red part in this case may not contain diagnostic tissue. This was a renal haemangiosarcoma and, as with splenic haemangiosarcoma, much of the centre was a haematoma, i.e. consisted of free blood that was not diagnostic in and of itself.

Renal haemangiosarcoma is a recognised, but much less common, form of visceral haemangiosarcoma in the dog. With respect to prognosis and likely behaviour of this particular subtype, there are more limited reports in the literature but progression does appear to be slower and survival times longer when compared to other forms of visceral haemangiosarcoma.[1]

> **TIP**
>
> If you have cases where you are uncertain if a lesion is neoplastic or inflammatory, it might be worth retaining a small portion of the other half fresh (chilled) for possible microbiology, in case this turned out not to be neoplastic. Freezing is less advisable as this can adversely affect the viability of certain pathogens.

## Reference

1  Locke, J. E., & Barber, L. G. (2006). Comparative aspects and clinical outcomes of canine renal hemangiosarcoma. *Journal of Veterinary Internal Medicine*, 20(4), 962–967. https://doi.org/10.1111/j.1939-1676.2006.tb01812.x

# URIN5 answers

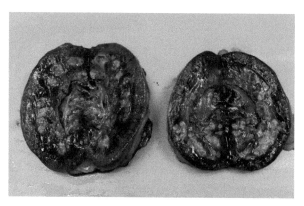

Fig. 6.5

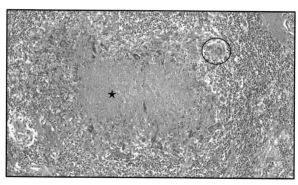

Fig. 6.6

## 1.    Describe any abnormalities in Fig. 6.5

On cut section, the cortex and medulla of both kidneys contain multifocal to coalescing, well-demarcated, yellow to pale tan, irregularly shaped and mostly non-raised lesions that range from 1 mm to 12 mm diameter. Some of these lesions are centrally cavitated (necrotic). The renal papilla (crest) is partially destroyed, with a slightly scalloped border, leading to mild pelvic dilation.

## 2.    Provide a diagnosis

Severe, bilateral, multifocal to coalescing, chronic, necrotising nephritis.

Pyelonephritis is also acceptable since the renal papilla is involved. The distribution is multifocal and bilateral, which supports haematogenous spread of an infectious agent to both kidneys. While some neoplasms can metastasise to the kidneys using this mechanism, the colour and central necrosis/cavitation in many of these lesions are more suggestive of an inflammatory, necrotising lesion, likely of infectious origin. In this case, histopathology was required to confirm that suspicion.

## 3.    Fig. 6.6 is a histopathological image of one of the lesions. The image does not contain any normal renal architecture. Identify the lesion, justify your reasoning and explain why there might be a health and safety concern with this case.

This is a centrally necrotic granuloma. The central pink necrotic area (*) is immediately surrounded by macrophages and multinucleated giant cells (circle) which are, in turn, rimmed by many plasma cells. *Mycobacterium* and fungal agents such as *Aspergillus fumigatus* are potential causes of necrosis and granulomatous inflammation, and both are potentially zoonotic, hence the health and safety risks (see Tip). Fig. 6.6a is a Gomori methanamine silver stain (GMS) used to highlight fungal organisms. In this case, the GMS confirms bilateral mycotic nephritis. *Aspergillus fumigatus* was cultured from the kidney.

---

### TIP – HEALTH AND SAFETY

Please do not forget potential zoonoses and protect yourself and your colleagues.

In general, necropsy facilities will have protocols for submission of samples potentially infected with mycobacterium, including cadavers (some may not accept suspect cases so it is always advisable to check with individual laboratories; it is likely they will have a specific protocol that you are asked to follow).

Suspect necropsies may be performed in a safety cabinet where cadaver size allows. Where this is not feasible, respiratory equipment is usually worn by all involved, in addition to routine personal protective equipment (waterproof coveralls, gloves, boots).

If you suspect a potentially zoonotic agent and do not have such facilities, you should not undertake the necropsy.

Culture of mycobacterium must be undertaken at an accredited laboratory and can take months as culture is slow. Molecular testing (PCR) is now more available, however, and can be undertaken on formalin-fixed tissue, although this is much less sensitive than fresh (~50% of positive cases are negative when conducted on fixed tissue).

Where infection is suspected (even if not, as you can still be caught out) retention of a fresh piece of tissue is prudent. This can be frozen for longer term storage, although this can affect viability of some organisms (generally not mycobacterium, which is quite robust).

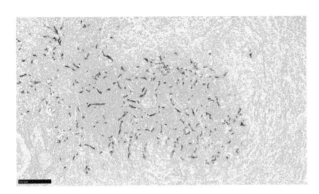

Fig. 6.6a

## Comment

German Shepherd Dogs are prone to disseminated Aspergillus infection. *Aspergillus fumigatus* is a potential cause but *A. terreus* and *A. deflectus* are more common. Clinical signs are dictated by the area of the body infected. When the kidneys are affected, which they commonly are, fungal hyphae can be detected in urine but more specific diagnostic tests are required to confirm the aetiology, particularly fungal culture. German Shepherds are also predisposed to immunoglobulin A (IgA) deficiency but, if there is a direct link between this deficiency and a predisposition to disseminated aspergillosis, it remains unproven.[1]

## Reference

1  Bennett, P. F., Talbot, J. J., Martin, P., Kidd, S. E., Makara, M., & Barrs, V. R. (2018). Long term survival of a dog with disseminated *Aspergillus deflectus* infection without definitive treatment. *Medical Mycology Case Reports*, *22*, 1–3. https://doi.org/10.1016/j.mmcr.2018.07.002

# URIN6 answers

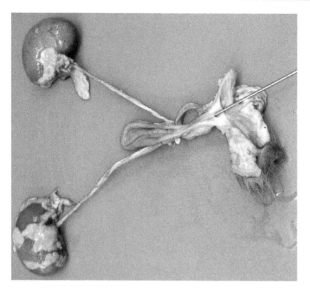

Fig. 6.7

## 1. Describe any abnormalities

The probe has been passed into the urethra and directly on into the lumen of one ureter without entering the urinary bladder lumen, indicating that the ureter is in the wrong position, i.e. ectopic.

## 2. Provide a diagnosis

Unilateral ectopic ureter.

## 3. Identify the relevant anatomic structures then compare your answer with Fig 6.7a (labelled)

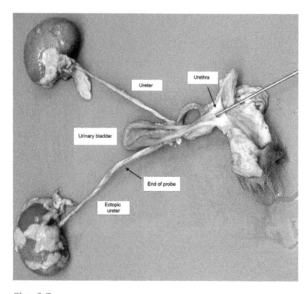

Fig. 6.7a

Ectopic ureter is a rare congenital anomaly that may be unilateral or bilateral.[1] In the dog, females are more commonly affected, although this may reflect the fact that affected females are usually incontinent from very early on in life (the demographics may also be skewed by underdiagnosis in males).[2] There are breed predilections, notably the Labrador and Golden retriever.[2] The condition may also be associated with other congenital anomalies of the urogenital tract.

> **TIP**
>
> If urinary incontinence is in the clinical history the best approach is to remove the urinary tract intact and in one piece.
>
> This allows retention of the normal relationships and permits passage of a probe to assess the route taken by the ureters.
>
> It is not enough just to follow the external path of the ureter. You must pass a probe into the lumen of the ureter and confirm whether or not it empties into the correct place, which is the trigone of the urinary bladder.

## References

1 Cianciolo, R. E., & Mohr, F. C. (2016). Urinary system. In M. G. Maxie (Ed.), *Jubb, Kennedy and Palmer's pathology of domestic animals* (6th ed), Vol. 2. Elsevier. https://doi.org/10.1016/B978-0-7020-5318-4.00010-3

2 Reichler, I. M., Eckrich Specker, C., Hubler, M., Boos, A., Haessig, M., & Arnold, S. (2012). Ectopic ureters in dogs: Clinical features, surgical techniques and outcome. *Veterinary Surgery, 41*(4), 515–522. https://doi.org/10.1111/j.1532-950X.2012.00952.x

# URIN7 answers

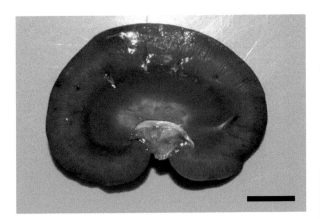

Fig. 6.8 Bar = 1 cm.

## 1.  Describe any abnormalities
There is a well-demarcated, irregular, yellow/orange lesion in the inner medulla and renal papilla, measuring approximately 13 mm × 3 mm. It is delineated by a thin red line which is in turn surrounded by a less well-demarcated, pale grey rim.

## 2.  Provide a diagnosis
Severe, diffuse, acute renal papillary necrosis.

## 3.  Link this lesion to the clinical history and briefly outline the pathogenesis
A key part of the history which is likely relevant is that the dog had received a non-steroidal anti-inflammatory drug (NSAID) in the weeks prior to the development of clinical signs. NSAIDs are a well-recognised cause of renal papillary necrosis. The mechanism centres on their inhibition of cyclooxygenase (COX). There are two types of COX: COX1, which is constitutive (i.e. essential to normal function), and COX2, which is only expressed during the inflammatory process. NSAIDs can inhibit both. COX1 is important in the production of prostaglandins, which are, in turn, key to the maintenance of vasodilation and blood flow to the renal tubules. Inhibition of this process leads to ischaemia and tubular necrosis, particularly in the renal papilla.

Renal papillary necrosis is not always a cause of death and it can be acute, subacute or even chronic. However, in its fulminant form, it can be fatal. It is usually bilateral but, in this case, the dog only had one kidney, which may have increased the clinical significance of the lesion.

---

TIP
- When sampling kidney, always make sure you sample cortex, medulla and renal papilla (crest). This case is a good example of why it is important to do this.
- Cut the kidney in half longitudinally. Place one-half on the cutting surface, flat side down and make a slice through it on the midline (see Fig. 6.8a). Make a parallel cut with the aim of creating a slice that is ~5–10 mm thick.
- Do the same for the other half and for the other kidney so that you have four sections.
- **Always** sample gross lesions too, of course!

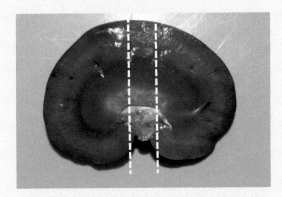

Fig. 6.8a Canine kidney. The two dashed lines indicate where to cut to obtain the best section for histopathology.

# URIN8 answers

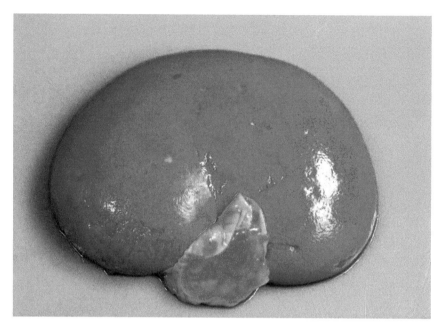

Fig. 6.9

## 1. Describe any abnormalities

The renal cortex is diffusely tan with a few irregular, ~1 mm diameter pitted lesions and a slightly granular surface (there is also a discrete, ~2 mm diameter, yellow focus on the cortex).

## 2. Provide a diagnosis

Severe diffuse acute tubular necrosis (acute kidney injury).

Acute tubular necrosis (also termed acute kidney injury[1]) is the most likely diagnosis and, in such cases, the cut surface of the cortex often bulges slightly. The canine kidney should normally be dark mahogany brown. Another differential to consider is infiltrative round cell neoplasia (although we would expect the kidney to be diffusely enlarged or multinodular; it would be unusual for infiltrative neoplasia in the kidney to be so uniform). Renal amyloidosis causes diffuse renal pallor but, due to deposition of amyloid, the kidney is usually uniformly enlarged and has a 'waxy' or turgid consistency. The discrete tan lesion may be an incidental, more chronic, pre-existing lesion but could also be a small cluster of inflammatory cells.

## 3. Given the clinical history, what is the most likely cause? List some other potential causes

Toxic injury and ischaemia are the two most likely causes of acute kidney injury but infection/inflammation may also be involved. There are many potentially nephrotoxic substances but broad categories include chemicals (e.g. oxalate crystals secondary to ethylene glycol ingestion); drugs (particularly antibiotics such as aminoglycosides; or non-steroidal anti-inflammatory drugs); pigments (haemoglobin, myoglobin); food substances (e.g. grapes, raisins, excess vitamin D); and infectious agents (*Leptospira*; *Babesia*; *Borrelia*).[1-3]

## References

1   Rimer, D., Chen, H., Bar-Nathan, M., & Segev, G. (2022). Acute kidney injury in dogs: Etiology, clinical and clinico-pathologic findings, prognostic markers, and outcome. *Journal of Veterinary Internal Medicine, 36*(2), 609–618. https://doi.org/10.1111/jvim.16375

2   Stokes, J. E., & Forrester, S. D. (2004). New and unusual causes of acute renal failure in dogs and cats. *Veterinary Clinics of North America. Small Animal Practice, 34*(4), 909–922. https://doi.org/10.1016/j.cvsm.2004.03.006

3   Schweighauser, A., Henke, D., Oevermann, A., Gurtner, C., & Francey, T. (2020). Toxicosis with grapes or raisins causing acute kidney injury and neurological signs in dogs. *Journal of Veterinary Internal Medicine, 34*(5), 1957–1966. https://doi.org/10.1111/jvim.15884

# URIN9 answers

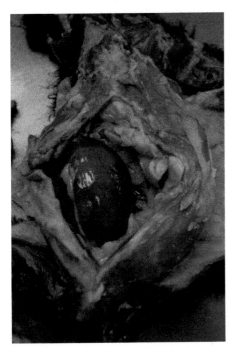

Fig. 6.10

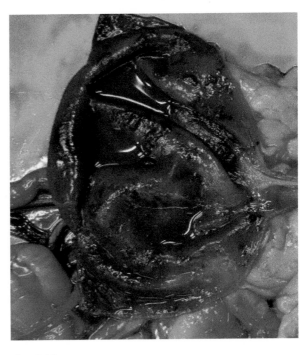

Fig. 6.11

### 1. Describe any abnormalities
This is the urinary bladder. It is markedly distended, thin-walled, turgid and diffusely discoloured and mottled red/purple to grey.

### 2. Provide a diagnosis
Severe urinary bladder distention with haemorrhage, ulceration and necrosis.

### 3. Where should you look next and why?
You should check the urethra along its entire length. This is the typical appearance of a urinary bladder from a blocked cat (i.e. due to urethral obstruction). The urine will also be dark red and contain clots of blood, and the bladder can rupture, which may lead to urine-induced peritonitis. Obstruction is usually due to uroliths (urinary calculi) or urethral plugs (a sludge-like material). If severe enough the damming back of urine may also distend the ureters and cause mucosal necrosis there too.

# URIN10 answers

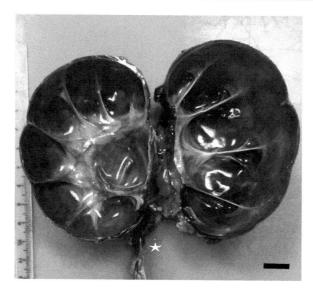

Fig. 6.12 **Bar = 1 cm.**

### 1.   Describe any abnormalities

There is virtually total loss of the cortical, medullary and papillary parenchyma with complete exposure of the calyces, due to marked, diffuse dilation of the renal pelvis. The kidney has effectively been turned into a thin-walled 'bag' of urine; on cut section it would have been full of urine. The proximal ureter is just visible – see white asterisk – it was moderately dilated.

### 2.   Provide a diagnosis

Severe unilateral hydronephrosis and moderate hydroureter.

### 3.   What is the underlying pathological process that leads to this lesion?

This lesion occurs due to pressure atrophy. Urine builds up due to blockage, leading to increased pressure proximal to the point of obstruction. Gradually, this pressure causes atrophy – through apoptosis – of the renal tissue. Other general (not specific to the kidney) types of pathological atrophy are (i) nutritional (ii) denervation (iii) hormonal [or lack of] (iv) disuse and (v) circulatory failure.

The contralateral kidney may be enlarged in such cases, due to compensatory hypertrophy. Hypertrophy is the opposite of atrophy, denoting enlargement of an organ (or individual cells). In this case the blockage was due to uroliths which is the most common trigger, but other causes include iatrogenic (i.e. ligature placement around a ureter at time of neutering); and a space-occupying lesion such as a neoplasm e.g. transitional cell carcinoma of the urinary bladder obstructing the ureter as it enters the bladder.

# URIN11 answers

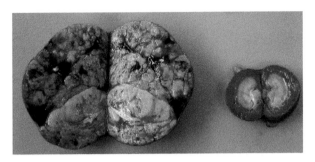

Fig. 6.13

## 1.   Describe any abnormalities

The left kidney is dramatically enlarged and the parenchyma is virtually completely replaced by a multilobulated, off-white/cream-coloured mass that bulges a little on cut section. There are multifocal dark red areas superimposed (haemorrhage). The right kidney is grossly normal.

## 2.   Provide a diagnosis

Renal carcinoma is most likely, given the gross appearance and age of the dog. This is the most common primary renal tumour in the dog, and it tends to be solitary and well-demarcated, often located in one of the poles of the affected kidney.[1]

Other primary renal neoplasms in the dog include adenoma, cystadenoma, cystadenocarcinoma, haemangioma, haemangiosarcoma and nephroblastoma. Urothelial tumours may arise in the renal pelvis but are rare. Adenomas are usually much smaller than this. Haemangiomas and haemangiosarcoma are usually dark red with much less solid substance – they often appear cystic or translucent. Nephroblastoma is a reasonable differential in this case, at least based on the gross appearance. However, it is generally a tumour of the juvenile dog, rather than the elderly, as in this case.

What about renal lymphoma? Primary renal lymphoma is believed to be rare in the dog, although the exact prevalence is unclear. Interestingly, primary renal lymphoma is typically bilateral.[2,3] It may present similarly to this case, with a bulging cut section, but would normally be whiter and more homogeneous. Metastatic lymphoma would, by definition, present with tumours in other organs and would be much more likely to present multifocally in both kidneys. The kidneys are prone to metastatic neoplasia and are often involved in any disseminated cancer. Other than lymphoma, examples of metastatic neoplasia include histiocytic sarcoma, haemangiosarcoma or metastatic carcinomas. This highlights the importance of a complete necropsy to exclude other potential sources of the cancer.

## 3.   How would you link the peritoneal effusion to the renal tumour in this case?

Renal carcinomas are able to invade the local vasculature, including the renal vein. They also have a high potential for metastasis. This may arise transcoelomically, i.e. directly onto the peritoneal surface, or via the vasculature to both kidneys, the lungs and liver. More distant metastasis can also occur (e.g. to the brain, lymph nodes and heart). Transcoelomic spread of tumour emboli may occur in some cases,[4] leading typically to blockage of lymphatic vessels and reduced drainage of abdominal fluid. Transcoelomic spread is otherwise known as carcinomatosis and is associated with a pronounced scirrhous reaction – the fibrous connective tissue in this reaction is more extensive and further impedes lymphatic drainage. This reaction occurs in several different types of carcinoma, including urothelial, pancreatic, prostatic and intestinal.

In cases where the carcinoma is solitary and has not appeared to spread or breach the renal capsule, total nephrectomy may be curative.

## References

1   Lucke, V. M., & Kelly, D. F. (1976). Renal carcinoma in the dog. *Veterinary Pathology*, *13*(4), 264–276. https://doi.org/10.1177/030098587601300403

2   Taylor, A., Finotello, R., Vilar-Saavedra, P., Couto, C. G., Benigni, L., & Lara-Garcia, A. (2019). Clinical characteristics and outcome of dogs with presumed primary renal lymphoma. *Journal of Small Animal Practice*, *60*(11), 663–670. https://doi.org/10.1111/jsap.13059

3   Snead, E. C. (2005). A case of bilateral renal lymphosarcoma with secondary polycythaemia and paraneoplastic syndromes of hypoglycaemia and uveitis in an English Springer Spaniel. *Veterinary and Comparative Oncology*, *3*(3), 139–144. https://doi.org/10.1111/j.1476-5810.2005.00069.x

4   Cianciolo, R. E., & Mohr, F. C. (2016). Urinary system. In M. G. Maxie (Ed.), *Jubb, Kennedy and Palmer's pathology of domestic animals* (6th ed), Vol. 2. Elsevier. https://doi.org/10.1016/B978-0-7020-5318-4.00010-3

# URIN12 answers

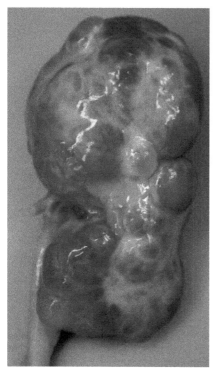

Fig. 6.14

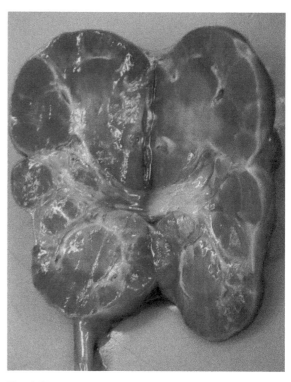

Fig. 6.15

## 1.   Describe any abnormalities

In Fig. 6.14 the kidney is severely misshapen with deep indentations and a very irregular profile. There are also several thin-walled cystic structures measuring up to approximately 1 cm diameter. The kidney is pale brown (much paler than normal in the dog), but the surface is partially obscured by grey/white bands and trabeculae of fibrous connective tissue.

Fig. 6.15 shows a longitudinal section through the kidney. There is still recognisable cortical and medullary architecture but the cortex is much paler than it should be and there are divisions resulting in increased nodularity, with formation of structures that have the appearance of separate small kidneys.

## 2.   Provide a diagnosis

Renal maldevelopment (dysplasia).

## 3.

(a)   Summarise the pertinent features of this condition in terms of pathogenesis and pathology.

Renal maldevelopment is a more recently introduced, and now preferred, term for renal dysplasia.[1] It is broadly used to describe chronic renal disease of early onset, usually in dogs less than two years of age. More specific terms are used for chronic nephropathies arising within particular breeds or families (e.g. familial nephropathy). An inherited basis has been proven in some of these breeds (e.g. familial glomerulonephropathy of the Bull Mastiff, which is almost certainly due to an autosomal recessive mode of inheritance[2]), but not all. Furthermore, nephropathies affecting litters may still be the result of environmental agents or infectious disease. In renal maldevelopment, the morphological features of affected kidneys are heterogenous and lesions may or may not be congenital. Microscopically, glomeruli and tubules may be involved and there will often be areas of immature glomeruli or a mismatch in the degree of maturity between different parts of the nephron.[3] When confronted with a young (or even not so young), pure breed dog in renal failure, at least consider the possibility of renal maldevelopment and bear in mind that some kidneys may only be smaller than normal – not necessarily as grossly distorted as in this case. The likelihood of a breed, familial or genetic basis increases if more than one or two dogs from the same background are affected. Breeds for which an inherited basis has been proven include the Bernese Mountain dog, Dalmatian, Bull Terrier, German Shepherd Dog, Irish Terrier, Norwegian Elkhound, Cairn Terrier and West Highland White Terrier, although some of these are still only suspected.[3]

Table 6.1 Non-renal lesions related to uraemia.[3]

| System | Lesion(s) | Mechanism |
|---|---|---|
| Alimentary | Ulceration (oral, especially ventrolateral tongue; stomach and intestine). May also see mineralisation of the gastric mucosa. | Uncertain – but related to vascular fibrinoid necrosis and elevated ammonia. |
| Respiratory | Alveolar mineralisation ('uraemic pneumonitis'). | Uncertain but may be related to imbalance in calcium and magnesium. |
| Muscle | Mineralisation of intercostal muscles. | Uncertain. |
| Endocrine | Hyperplasia of both parathyroid glands. | Low serum calcium levels trigger hyperplasia with the ultimate aim of increasing parathyroid hormone. This facilitates osteoclastic resorption of bone and stabilises calcium. |
| Skeleton | Fibrous osteodystrophy ('rubber jaw'). | This may be the result of excessive action of parathyroid hormone. It manifests most severely in the flat bones of the skull. |
| Central nervous system | Spongiform degeneration in the white matter ('uraemic encephalopathy'). | Uncertain. |
| Connective tissues | Soft tissue mineralisation. | Likely due to hypercalcaemia since, in renal disease, serum calcium may be abnormally low or high. |

(b)   Provide at least **FIVE** grossly appreciable necropsy lesions you might expect to find associated with the clinical diagnosis of uraemia.

Helpful flags of uraemia at gross necropsy are myriad but they do not usually all occur concurrently – we may only see one or two (or none) in any one animal – and some are very uncommon. However, the main ones are outlined in Table 6.1.

---

TIP: URAEMIA VERSUS AZOTAEMIA[3]

Do not confuse these two terms. Azotaemia is defined as elevated nitrogen containing chemicals in the blood, notably urea and creatinine. It is a biochemical abnormality and may be the result of reduced perfusion of the kidneys, e.g. due to dehydration, shock or heart failure (prerenal azotaemia); kidney failure (renal azotaemia); or obstruction of urine outflow (postrenal).

Uraemia also implies increased urea in the blood stream but specifically due to renal failure. The term is used, however, to describe a clinical syndrome of renal failure which may include lesions in organs and tissues external to the kidneys.

---

## References

1   Cianciolo, R., Brown, C., Mohr, C., Nabity, M., Van der Lugt, J., McLeland, S., Aresu, L., Benali, S., Spangler, B., Amerman, H. et al. (2018). *Atlas of renal lesions in proteinuric dogs.* Ohio State University Press. https://ohiostate.pressbooks.pub/vetrenalpathatlas/

2   Casal, M. L., Dambach, D. M., Meister, T., Jezyk, P. F., Patterson, D. F., & Henthorn, P. S. (2004). Familial glomerulonephropathy in the bull mastiff. *Veterinary Pathology*, 41(4), 319–325. https://doi.org/10.1354/vp.41-4-319

3   Cianciolo, R. E., & Mohr, F. C. (2016). Urinary system. In M. G. Maxie (Ed.), *Jubb, Kennedy and Palmer's pathology of domestic animals* (6th ed), Vol. 2. Elsevier. https://doi.org/10.1016/B978-0-7020-5318-4.00010-3

# Musculoskeletal cases

7

# MS1

## Topics

- Prioritisation of findings
- Approach to difficult cases
- Generation of pathological differential diagnoses lists
- Practical technique

## History

A 9Y old, male neutered Boxer presented for necropsy following euthanasia due to hind limb weakness that had begun 18 months previously. There was very little response to empirical therapy and the paresis eventually progressed to hind limb paralysis and proprioceptive ataxia. The dog was otherwise alert and eating well. Vaccination history was complete and there was no history of travel outside the United Kingdom. Haematology and a basic panel of biochemistry were within normal limits, other than mild and persistently elevated creatine kinase (CK). Hind limb and thoracolumbar spine radiographs were normal but there was mildly elevated protein in the cerebrospinal fluid. There was no history of trauma.

## Questions

1. List some differential diagnoses you might consider prior to beginning the necropsy.
2. Outline how you would approach sampling of skeletal muscle in a dog, whether during necropsy or as a surgical biopsy. How would you prepare the sample(s) for submission to a pathology laboratory?

# MS2

## Topic

Lesion recognition

## History

This was one of several gross lesions in a 12Y old, Gordon Setter that had died due to severe haemorrhage from a splenic haemangiosarcoma.

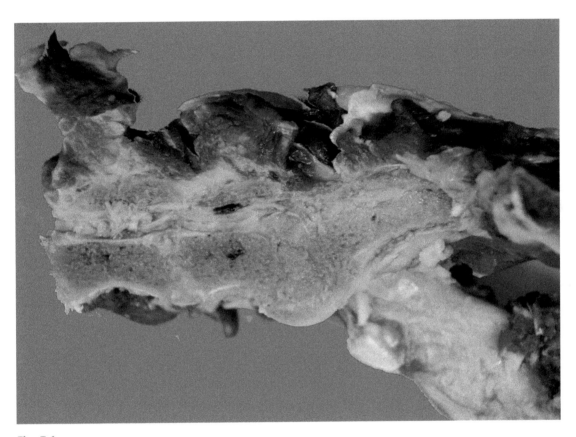

Fig. 7.1

## Questions

1. Describe any abnormalities.
2. Provide a diagnosis.
3. What is the clinical significance of this lesion?

# MS3

## Topics

**Lesion recognition**

**Prioritisation of findings**

**Pathogenesis**

## History

This vertebral column was collected at necropsy from a middle-aged, male bush dog with a history of progressive hind limb paresis and back pain.

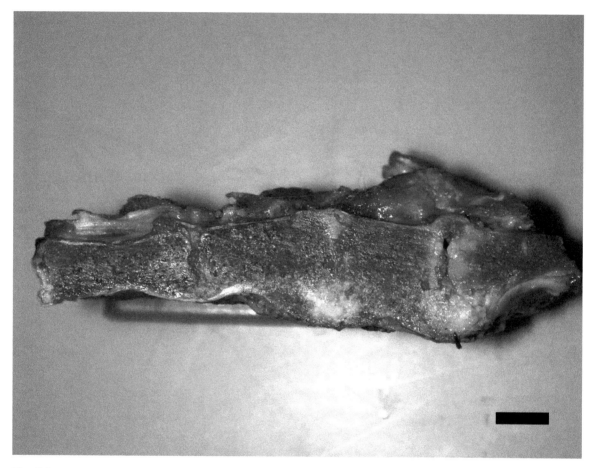

Fig. 7.2

## Questions

1. Describe any abnormalities.
2. Provide a diagnosis.
3. How does the pathogenesis of this condition differ between, for example, an ageing Labrador and a young Dachshund?

# MS4

## Topics

Lesion recognition

Pathogenesis

## History

Figs 7.3 (left hip) and 7.4 (right hip) illustrate incidental necropsy findings in a 10Y old, male Old English Sheepdog that was euthanised due to multicentric neoplasia.

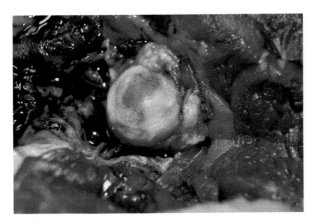

Fig. 7.3

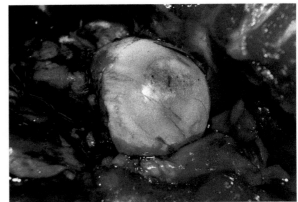

Fig 7.4

## Questions

1. Describe any abnormalities.
2. Provide a diagnosis.
3. The exposed subchondral bone is very smooth and shiny, an effect known as 'eburnation'. What does eburnation mean?

# MS5

## Topics

Lesion recognition

Pathogenesis

## History

This was a necropsy finding in a 9Y old, female neutered Labrador that had died as a result of acute pancreatitis.

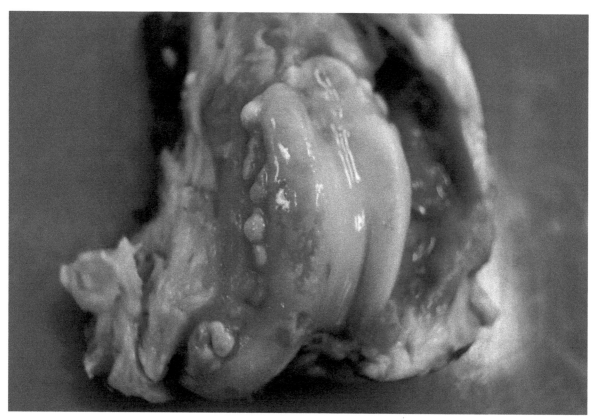

Fig. 7.5

## Questions

1. Describe any abnormalities.
2. Provide a diagnosis.
3. Outline some possible causes of this lesion.

# MS6

## Topics

**Lesion recognition**

**Pathogenesis**

## History

This 5Y old, male neutered cat had presented for veterinary attention after being found at the side of the road having been hit by a car. It died as treatment was being pursued, by which time its owners had been found. They requested a necropsy.

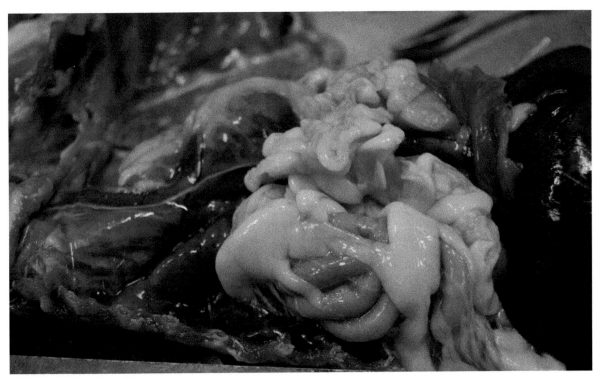

Fig. 7.6

## Questions

1. Describe any abnormalities.
2. Provide a diagnosis.
3. Outline the potential pathogenesis of this lesion **AND** the likely cause of death.

# MS7

## Topics

Practical technique

Lesion recognition

Approach to difficult cases

## History

A 9Y old, female neutered Rottweiler was euthanised after a lytic and mildly proliferative bone lesion was found in the right proximal humerus (the dog's right hind limb had been removed one year previously). The gross appearance of the lesion is illustrated in Figs 7.7 and 7.8.

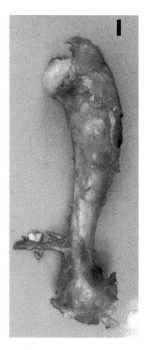

Fig. 7.7 **Bar = 1 cm.**

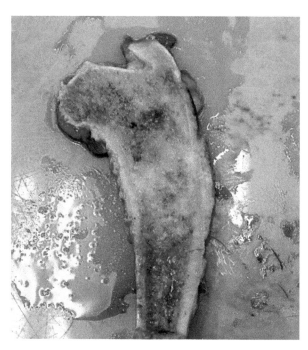

Fig. 7.8

## Questions

1. Describe any abnormalities.
2. Provide a diagnosis.
3. Name the **THREE** other predisposed sites in the dog, and the likely biological behaviour of this lesion.

# MS1 answers

## 1.   List some differential diagnoses you might consider prior to beginning the necropsy

The clinical presentation and history suggest nervous or musculoskeletal disease so the differentials are potentially myriad. Hind limb weakness progressing to paralysis is particularly supportive of spinal cord disease. Mildly elevated CK levels could be secondary to the hind limb weakness – one would expect CK levels to be more substantially elevated in a primary myositis, myopathy or muscular dystrophy.

Main differentials for slowly progressive hind limb weakness in an older dog are the following.

1. Neoplasia: This category can be further divided into extradural (external to the dura mater), intradural/extramedullary (between the parenchyma and the dura) and intramedullary (within the cord parenchyma) neoplasia. There are numerous possible differentials and many forms of neoplasia are rare.[1–3] The majority arise external to the dura mater and include neoplastic processes involving bone, myeloid tissue, cartilage and other connective tissues (e.g. lymphoma, haemangiosarcoma, multiple myeloma, osteosarcoma, and liposarcoma), as well as metastatic neoplasms (e.g. metastatic carcinoma, metastatic haemangiosarcoma, malignant melanoma). It is much less common to see intradural tumours or tumours within the cord itself but this category includes meningiomas, nerve sheath tumours and gliomas.[3]

2. Degenerative disease, particularly intervertebral disc disease but consider also degenerative myelopathy or peripheral neuropathy.

3. Severe degenerative joint disease (osteoarthritis) in the hind limbs.

4. Infectious myelitis or spinal meningitis: This may be due to viral (e.g. distemper), bacterial, fungal (less likely in the UK) or protozoal disease. Neospora caninum is an important differential for hind limb weakness but is a disease of very young dogs, usually manifesting clinically from 3–8 weeks of age.

5. Non-infectious spinal diseases: Examples include steroid-responsive meningitis-arteritis (previously variously known as steroid-responsive meningitis, Beagle pain syndrome and juvenile polyarteritis)[4] and meningoencephalomyelitis of unknown origin, which includes granulomatous meningoencephalitis (GME).[5]

6. Primary muscle disease (myopathy or myositis), most notably polymyositis (which may be immune mediated or infectious, due to *N. caninum* or *Toxoplasma gondii*).

7. Other differentials such as ischaemia or infarction (e.g. saddle thrombus, fibrocartilaginous embolic myelopathy) are unlikely as they would typically present more acutely, usually without further progression. Similarly, congenital disease is unlikely to appear at this stage in life.

## 2.   Outline how you would approach sampling of skeletal muscle in a dog, whether during necropsy or as a surgical biopsy. How would you prepare the sample(s) for submission to a pathology laboratory?

A sensible approach when taking surgical biopsy muscle samples is outlined below.

1. Collect fresh and formalin-fixed samples from a forelimb muscle, a hindlimb muscle and a muscle of mastication.

2. Each sample should measure 5 mm × 5 mm × 10 mm where feasible.

3. One sample from each site is fixed in 10% neutral buffered formalin. The sample can be (gently) sutured or stapled to a flat wooden stick (lollipop stick, tongue depressor) to prevent hypercontraction during fixation. However, stapling (and even the stick) may not be necessary. Seal the formalin container in a zip lock bag.

4. One sample from each site should be submitted fresh. To do this, wrap the muscle sample in damp gauze (not soaking wet) then place in a plastic container. The container should be placed close to an ice pack but not touching – it is best to insulate the container and ice pack with bubble wrap and place in a zip lock bag. Different samples should be in separate containers.

5. **ALWAYS** include signalment and a concise clinical history. Particularly helpful clinical information is:
   a. main presenting signs (e.g. weakness, exercise intolerance, any respiratory signs or regurgitation).
   b. age of onset and pattern of development (e.g. progressive, intermittent, waxing and waning).
   c. results of other diagnostic tests (especially creatine kinase levels; any serology (e.g. *T. gondii*, type IIM antibodies).
   d. Which muscles have been biopsied.

## Sampling during necropsy

The obvious advantage of sampling muscle at necropsy is that multiple muscles can be sampled and there is no restriction in terms of size of sample and access to it. Similar sites can be sampled, as for surgical biopsies, but further sites can be sampled as dictated by clinical signs. Other samples that can be easily included at necropsy are: Oesophagus (some forms of muscle disease involve the oesophageal muscle, notably polymyositis); diaphragm; tongue; and heart (although heart is more likely to be involved in farm animal muscle diseases such as white muscle disease and blackleg). It is worth retaining fresh, frozen muscle, as well as formalin-fixed muscle. The images below detail how to take a muscle sample at necropsy.

Note: If you ever have need to send fresh muscle to a laboratory, do not send it on cardboard as this will desiccate the muscle. It is always best to follow the laboratory's advice but, in most cases, sending fresh muscle wrapped in moist gauze in a clean universal container next to an ice pack (and insulated from the ice pack by bubble wrap or similar) will be the best approach.

The final diagnosis in this case was degenerative myelopathy. This is a slowly progressive disease that occurs in many breeds of dog, notably the German Shepherd Dog. However, the Boxer is also disproportionately affected.

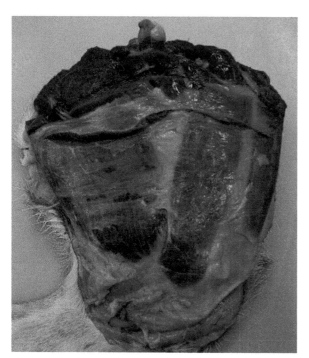

Fig. 7.9 **Step 1:** Strip the skin from an area such as the medial thigh where it is easiest to access long lengths of muscle.

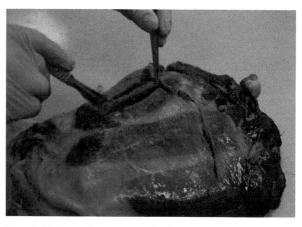

Fig. 7.10 **Step 2:** Use a scalpel to make parallel incisions in the muscle that run in the same direction as the long axis of the myofibres ('with the grain'). Do not worry too much about dimensions at this stage as you can trim further before fixing.

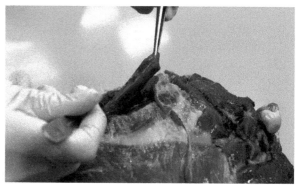

Fig. 7.11 **Step 3:** Grasp the muscle sample at one end and try not to move the forceps from that end. This will restrict any crush artefact to one small area of the sample and can be trimmed off.
  Aim to take a sample that is approximately 5 cm long, with the other two dimensions measuring no more than 1 cm.

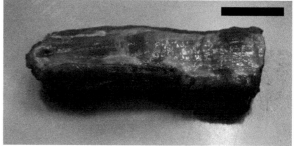

Fig. 7.12 **Step 4:** Place the muscle on a cutting board and trim any crushed areas from the ends. Make sure that at least one dimension measures no more than 1 cm. This can be placed on cardboard prior to fixing but we find this is not absolutely necessary. We also prefer to avoid suturing or stapling the muscle to card as this can lead to handling artefacts.

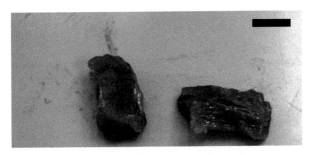

**Fig. 7.13** Step 5: The muscle is trimmed after fixation but these two sections illustrate the sections that are best evaluated histologically – one transverse and one longitudinal. This is why we take a long sample rather than a cube – to allow for both planes of section to be processed. These planes complement each other in the structural information they can provide. For instance, denervation atrophy is best assessed in transverse sections and regeneration in longitudinal sections.

Most cases are euthanised on welfare grounds, but clinical signs include upper motor neuron paresis, proprioceptive ataxia, exaggerated pelvic limb spinal reflexes and, ultimately, incontinence.[6] The diagnosis is a histological one. Lesions comprise Wallerian-type degeneration (myelin vacuolation, axonal degeneration and myelomacrophages) with astrocytosis, primarily in the thoracolumbar segments (T3-L3). The condition is genetic, caused by a mutation in the gene encoding the anti-oxidant enzyme superoxide dismutase.[7]

## References

1   Smith, A. N. (2020). Neoplasia of the nervous system in animals. *MSD Veterinary Manual.* msdvetmanual.com

2   Pancotto, T. E., Rossmeisl, Jr., J. H., Zimmerman, K., Robertson, J. L., & Werre, S. R. (2013). Intramedullary spinal cord neoplasia in 53 dogs (1990–2010): Distribution, clinicopathologic characteristics, and clinical behavior. *Journal of Veterinary Internal Medicine, 27*(6), 1500–1508. https://doi.org/10.1111/jvim.12182

3   Rissi, D. R., Barber, R., Burnum, A., & Miller, A. D. (2017). Canine spinal cord glioma. *Journal of Veterinary Diagnostic Investigation, 29*(1), 126–132. https://doi.org/10.1177/1040638716673127

4   Tipold, A., & Schatzberg, S. J. (2010). An update on steroid responsive meningitis-arteritis. *Journal of Small Animal Practice, 51*(3), 150–154. https://doi.org/10.1111/j.1748-5827.2009.00848.x

5   Coates, J. R., & Jeffery, N. D. (2014). Perspectives on meningoencephalomyelitis of unknown origin. *Veterinary Clinics of North America. Small Animal Practice, 44*(6), 1157–1185. https://doi.org/10.1016/j.cvsm.2014.07.009

6   Miller, A. D., Barber, R., Porter, B. F., Peters, R. M., Kent, M., Platt, S. R., & Schatzberg, S. J. (2009). Degenerative myelopathy in two boxer dogs. *Veterinary Pathology, 46*(4), 684–687. https://doi.org/10.1354/vp.08-VP-0270-M-BC

7   Shelton, G. D., Johnson, G. C., O'Brien, D. P., Katz, M. L., Pesayco, J. P., Chang, B. J., Mizisin, A. P., & Coates, J. R. (2012). Degenerative myelopathy associated with a missense mutation in the superoxide dismutase 1 (SOD1) gene progresses to peripheral neuropathy in Pembroke Welsh Corgis and Boxers. *Journal of the Neurological Sciences, 318*(1–2), 55–64. https://doi.org/10.1016/j.jns.2012.04.003

# MS2 answers

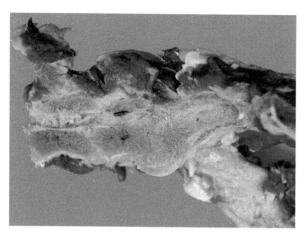

Fig. 7.1

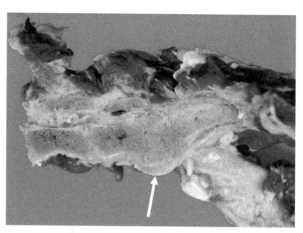

Fig. 7.1a Canine vertebral column with ankylosing spondylosis (white arrow).

### 1. Describe any abnormalities

The lesion comprises a focal, smooth-bordered proliferation of hard, fawn to white material (bone) on the ventral aspect of the caudal vertebral column, in line with the intervertebral space. This bone is essentially a large osteophyte and, in this case, forms a bridge between adjacent vertebrae. See Fig. 7.1a.

### 2. Provide a diagnosis

Ankylosing spondylosis.

### 3. What is the clinical significance of this lesion?

The clinical significance is generally negligible since there are often no clincial signs. However, it can be associated with stiffness and discomfort in the back. This particular lesion has formed in the lumbosacral region but, in dogs, another common site is in the area of the first two lumbar vertebrae.

Ankylosing spondylosis arises due to intervertebral disc degeneration, specifically degeneration and displacement of the annulus fibrosus, which triggers bone formation along the ventral margin of the intervertberal disc. It is important to look for evidence of intervertebral disc protrusion too when you see this lesion.

# MS3 answers

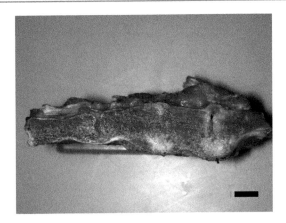

Fig. 7.2

## 1.  Describe any abnormalities

The sample comprises four vertebral bodies and their intervertebral discs. In the two discs on the right side of the image there is collapse of the intervertebral space and dorsal prolapse of the disc material, manifesting as two white nodules that bulge into the overlying spinal canal. Ventral to the same disc spaces there are two slightly larger, ill-defined, white nodules (approximately 1 cm diameter), resulting in distortion of the vertebral column's ventral profile (see Fig. 7.2a).

## 2.  Provide a diagnosis

Severe multifocal intervertebral disc degeneration with prolapse and ankylosing spondylosis.

In other words, this is intervertebral disc disease (IVDD). In Fig. 7.2a the lesions annotated by the arrows comprise degenerate intervertebral discs that have prolapsed into the spinal canal. They are the most significant lesions in the image since prolapse often causes spinal cord compression, accounting for the clinical signs in this case. There are two types of disc herniation, Hansen type I and Hansen type II. Type II herniations are partial, while type I herniations are complete, with rupture of the annulus fibrosus and

rapid propulsion of disc material into the vertebral canal. The lesions depicted by the asterisks are consistent with ankylosing spondylosis.

## 3.  How does the pathogenesis of this condition differ between, for example, an ageing Labrador and a young Dachshund?

Dachshunds fall into the chondrodystrophic category of dog breed (others include the Basset Hound, Pekingese, Beagle, Poodle and Corgi). They are prone to early onset chondroid degeneration of the nucleus pulposus. The degenerate nucleus mineralises and crumbles. The annulus fibrosus undergoes secondary degeneration and tears, allowing the disc material to prolapse. Since the annulus fibrosus is twice as thick ventrally as it is dorsally, prolapse is usually in a dorsal direction. These cases typically occur in younger dogs. The Labrador is a non-chondrodystrophic breed and disc degeneration is age related. Degenerative changes arise in both the annulus fibrosus and nucleus pulposus. In such cases, the nucleus is replaced by fibrocartilaginous tissue secondary to proteoglycan degradation and loss.

Refer to case MS2 for more information on ankylosing spondylosis.

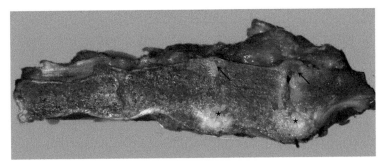

Fig. 7.2a Degenerative intervertebral disc disease and ankylosis, bush dog. There is prolapse of degenerate disc material at two sites (arrows) – they are protruding into the spinal canal and would have been associated with cord compression. The asterisks denote the areas of ankylosing spondylosis in the ventral surface of the vertebral column.

# MS4 answers

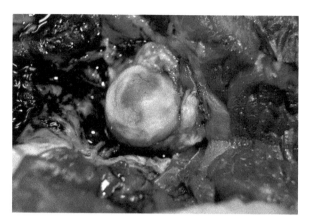

Fig. 7.3

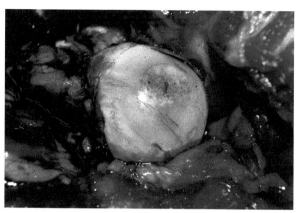

Fig. 7.4

### 1.    Describe any abnormalities

There is marked thinning, red/brown discolouration and roughening of the articular cartilage over the central part of the right femoral head, affecting approximately 50% of the surface area. There is similar loss of central cartilage from the left femoral head, though this is complete thickness with exposure of subchondral bone. The exposed bone has a very smooth and shiny appearance. When evaluating joint surfaces it can be helpful to gently tap the surface with the back of the blade to hear the different tone elicited from the intact cartilage (dull tone) and exposed bone (sharper tone with a slightly higher pitch), similar to the difference between tapping the pad of your finger versus your nail on a desk.

### 2.    Provide a diagnosis

Severe bilateral degenerative joint disease (DJD) – coxofemoral joints.

### 3.    The exposed subchondral bone is very smooth and shiny, an effect known as 'eburnation'. What does eburnation mean?

Eburnation is a degenerative change that implies polishing of exposed subchondral bone over a period of time, such that it becomes very dense and sclerotic, resembling ivory. Although this was an incidental finding in this case, it indicates severe, longstanding DJD, and the exposure of subchondral bone would have been painful. Note that DJD is a synonym for osteoarthritis.

# MS5 answers

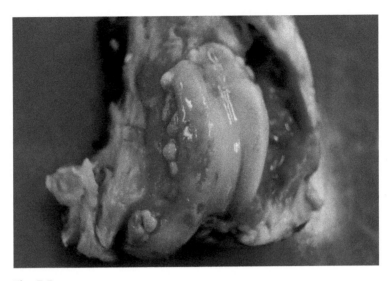

Fig. 7.5

## 1.   Describe any abnormalities

Along the borders of the femoral condyles and trochlear ridges (medial is most visible) there are multiple, raised, smooth, off-white/pale pink nodules that sometimes coalesce and range in diameter up to approximately 5 mm. There is a rusty brown, linear area of articular cartilage loss on the medial condyle. The synovial lining is also discoloured rusty brown.

## 2.   Provide a diagnosis

Degenerative joint disease (DJD) with multiple osteophytes

## 3.   Outline some possible causes of this lesion

DJD is also known as osteoarthritis. It may be primary (i.e. idiopathic although likely due to ageing) or secondary and may affect only one joint or multiple joints. Most likely, it reflects a common end stage for many different triggering causes. Secondary DJD may be due to previous inflammation (infectious or immune-mediated arthritis) or trauma (e.g. ruptured cruciate ligament) but joint instability is an important underlying reason and that may be conformational, with DJD developing as the animal gets older and the joint is subjected to abnormal or excessive stresses and strains.

The rusty brown discolouration is more unusual in this case but is a recognised associated change. It is most likely due to previous haemorrhage (i.e. haemosiderin pigmentation resulting from breakdown of haemoglobin). We also hypothesise that it may be partly due to deposition of lipofuscin or ceroid, cell membrane breakdown products that cause brown tingeing of the soft tissues. Lipofuscin is an ageing pigment that is composed of lipids and proteins but originates from cell membranes damaged by oxidation. Ceroid is broadly similar though some consider it to be solely associated with pathological processes.[1]

## Reference

1   Seehafer, S. S., & Pearce, D. A. (2006). You say lipofuscin, we say ceroid: Defining autofluorescent storage material. *Neurobiology of Aging*, *27*(4), 576–588. https://doi.org/10.1016/j.neurobiolaging.2005.12.006

# MS6 answers

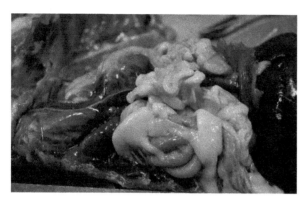

Fig. 7.6

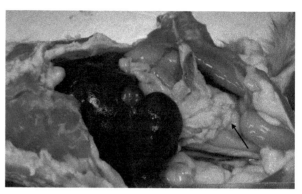

Fig. 7.6b **Feline abdominal cavity.** This illustrates the necropsy findings prior to opening the thoracic cavity. The loops of intestine in the abdominal cavity comprise large intestine only and you can appreciate some slight tension on the intestinal tract (black arrow) as a result of the cranial displacement of most of the small intestine.

### 1.  Describe any abnormalities

Virtually the entire small intestine occupies the mid to caudal thoracic cavity (review Fig. 7.6a for orientation if required). Not visible in the image was a tear in the diaphragm with associated haemorrhage. The intestinal loops also appear moderately dilated for a cat.

### 2.  Provide a diagnosis

Diaphragmatic tear with herniation of small intestine.

### 3.  Outline the potential pathogenesis of this lesion **AND** the likely cause of death

Diaphragmatic hernias are typically of traumatic origin, arising secondary to blunt trauma such as a road traffic accident, fall from a height or other significant abdominal trauma. The history in this case would tend to support that, along with the associated haemorrhage. The other main cause is a congenital hernia caused by weakening of the diaphragm.

Cause of death is most likely respiratory insufficiency leading to hypoxia. However, shock may have contributed, particularly cardiovascular shock.

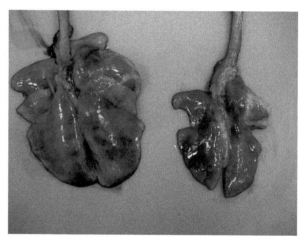

Fig. 7.6c **These two sets of lungs are from two other unrelated cases. Those on the left are normal, other than some postmortem discolouration, but those on the right are from another cat with a diaphragmatic hernia. They are collapsed as a result of the herniation.**

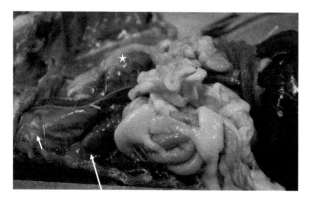

Fig. 7.6a **Feline thoracic cavity with herniated intestines. Heart (white asterisk); right cranial lung lobe (long arrow); thymic remnant (short arrow).**

# MS7 answers

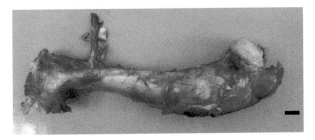

Fig. 7.7  **Bar = 1 cm.**

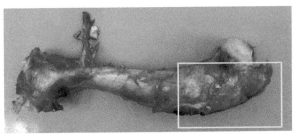

Fig. 7.7a

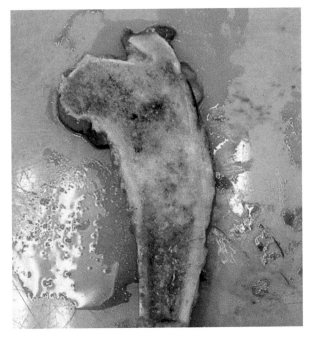

Fig. 7.8

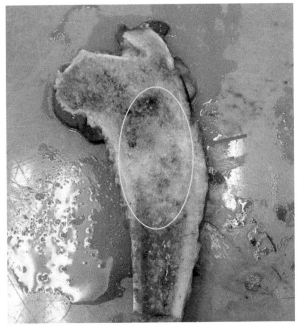

Fig. 7.8a

## 1.  Describe any abnormalities

Fig 7.7: There is an ill-defined, pale yellow, irregular, periosteal swelling distal to the humeral head, spanning an area measuring ~5 cm × 3 cm. Note, this swelling was hard grossly. See Fig. 7.7a, yellow box.

Fig 7.8: On cut section, corresponding to the swollen area in Fig. 7.7, the medulla is focally effaced by slightly bulging, pale yellow material (Fig. 7.8a, yellow oval). The cortex is also thickened (see Fig. 7.8a, red arrow).

## 2.  Provide a diagnosis

Appendicular osteosarcoma. An osteosarcoma is defined as a malignant mesenchymal tumour that produces bone. Most arise in the skeleton, and the proximal humerus is a predisposed site in the dog.

## 3.  Name the **THREE** other predisposed sites in the dog, and the likely biological behaviour of this lesion

Predisposed sites: Distal radius; distal femur; proximal tibia ('away from the elbow; towards the knee').

Behaviour: This is an aggressive malignancy that has often metastasised by the time the diagnosis is made. Metastasis occurs to the lungs but other visceral organs may become involved (e.g. kidneys) and mestastasis can also occur to other bones. Fig. 7.8b is an image of a metastatic deposit of osteosarcoma in the cerebrum of a different canine case. However, one study has reported an increased risk of brain metastasis in Rottweilers with appendicular osteosarcoma.[1]

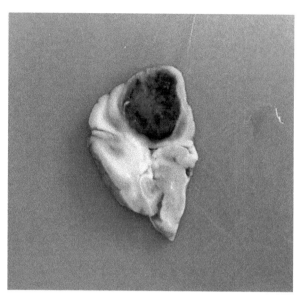

**Fig. 7.8b** Metastatic osteosarcoma, canine cerebrum.

## Reference

1   McNeill, C. J., Overley, B., Shofer, F. S., Kent, M. S., Clifford, C. A., Samluk, M., Haney, S., Van Winkle, T. J., & Sorenmo, K. U. (2007). Characterisation of the biological behaviour of appendicular osteosarcoma in Rottweilers and a comparison with other breeds: A review of 258 dogs. *Veterinary and Comparative Oncology*, *5*(2), 90–98. https://doi.org/10.1111/j.1476-5829.2006.00116.x

> **TIP**
>
> It can sometimes be difficult to identify bone lesions grossly, even tumours, particularly in earlier stages or if secondary lesions such as bone proliferation and lysis are subtle.
>
> Access to clinical images is extremely helpful so always try to obtain these if possible.
>
> Take the entire affected bone and, if there is a contralateral bone, compare to that.
>
> Always section the bone at time of necropsy using a saw. This will allow evaluation of the medulla and the cortical thickness.
>
> If you cannot see anything grossly, take lots of representative samples and retain the affected bone in formalin. It is often the case that even subtle macroscopic lesions are much more rewarding histologically so it is well worth taking plenty of sections for histopathology.

# Haematopoietic cases

8

# HAEM1

## Topics

**Lesion recognition**

**Generation of pathological differential diagnoses lists**

**Integration of pathological findings with clinical aspects**

## History

Necropsy finding in a 3Y old, male neutered Cocker Spaniel with a history of icterus. The liver was grossly and histologically normal, and there was no evidence of bile duct obstruction.

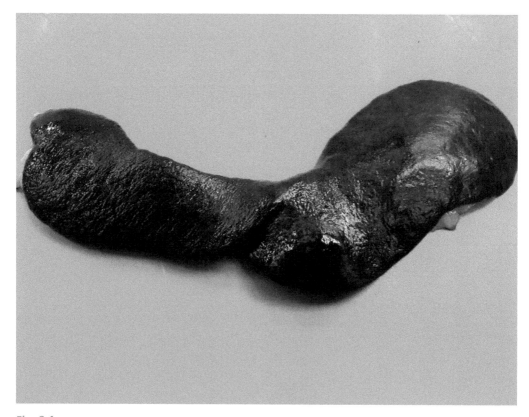

Fig. 8.1

## Questions

1. Describe any abnormalities.
2. Provide a diagnosis.
3. Provide some potential underlying causes for this lesion and suggest how you might link this lesion to the icterus.

# HAEM2

## Topics

Lesion recognition

Generation of pathological differential diagnoses lists

Pathogenesis

Health and safety

## History

A 4Y old, female spayed Springer Spaniel was necropsied following a short illness comprising lethargy and weakness.

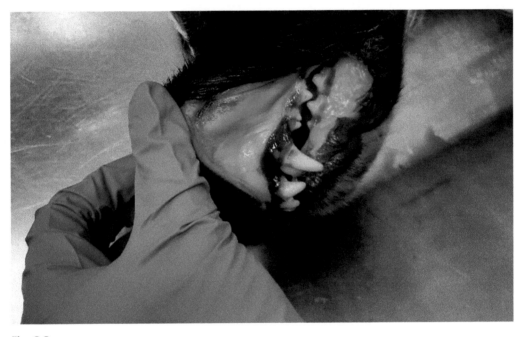

Fig. 8.2

## Questions

1. Describe any abnormalities.
2. Provide a diagnosis.
3. Outline the main potential causes of this condition, taking into considering any health and safety implications.

# HAEM3

## Topics

Lesion recognition

Prioritisation of findings

Generation of pathological differential diagnoses lists

Practical technique

## History

Fig. 8.3 illustrates an additional necropsy finding in a 7Y old, male neutered Doberman Pinscher that died due to a cardiomyopathy.

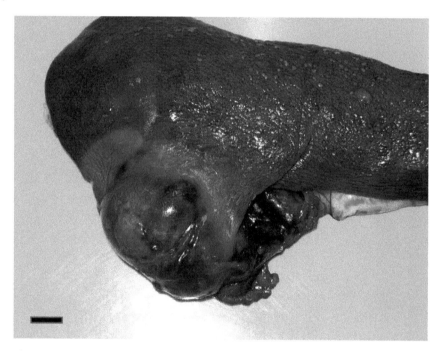

Fig. 8.3

## Questions

1. Describe any abnormalities.
2. Provide a diagnosis.
3. What is the clinical significance of any lesion(s) identified?

# HAEM4

## Topics

Lesion recognition

Generation of pathological differential diagnoses lists

## History

A 3Y old, female Springer Spaniel was euthanised after a long period of anorexia, weight loss and vomiting with no response to treatment.

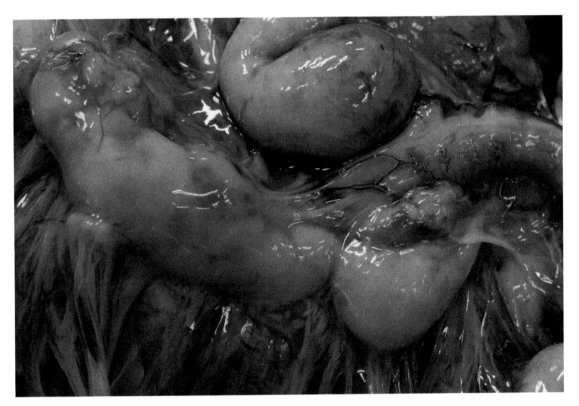

Fig. 8.4

## Questions

1. Describe any abnormalities.
2. Provide a diagnosis.
3. Outline some differential diagnoses.

# HAEM5

## Topics

**Lesion recognition**

**Generation of pathological differential diagnoses lists**

## History

A 10Y old, female neutered German Shepherd Dog presented for necropsy following euthanasia, having initially presented with exercise intolerance, deteriorating to respiratory distress. A cranial thoracic mass was detected radiographically.

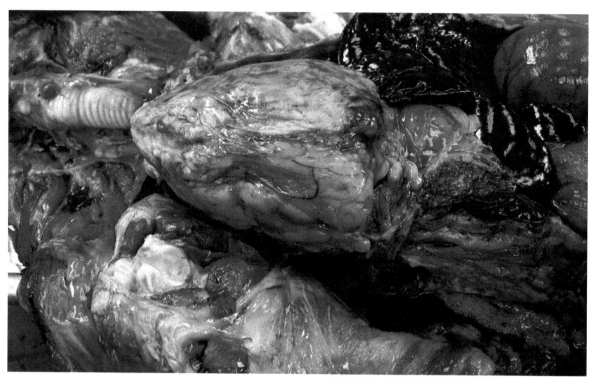

Fig. 8.5

## Questions

1. Describe any abnormalities.
2. Provide a diagnosis.
3. a) Name at least **TWO** conditions or other lesions associated with your diagnosis in the dog.
   b) List some other differentials for a mass within the cranial thoracic cavity.

# HAEM6

## Topics

Lesion recognition

Generation of pathological differential diagnoses lists

Pathogenesis

## History

A 10-week-old, male Border Collie puppy presented for necropsy after a two-week period of vomiting and diarrhoea that ultimately led to its death, despite empirical treatment. One of the main gross findings is shown in Fig. 8.6.

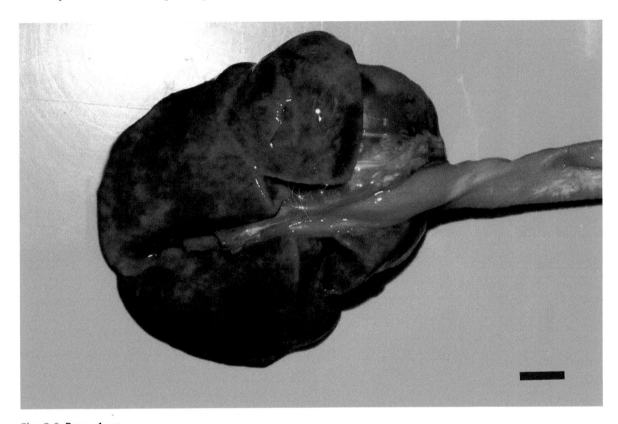

Fig. 8.6 Bar = 1 cm.

## Questions

1. Describe any abnormalities.
2. Provide a diagnosis.
3. Based on the history, outline some differential diagnoses and the possible pathogenesis of this lesion.

# HAEM7

## Topics

Lesion recognition

Common artefacts and pitfalls

Integration of pathological findings with clinical aspects

## History

Fig. 8.7 is from an 8Y old, male neutered Weimaraner that was necropsied after it died in transit during relocation from abroad.

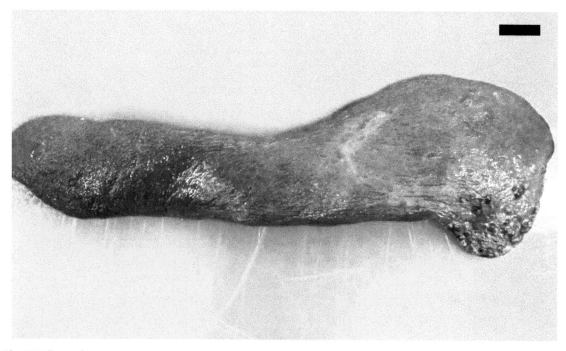

Fig. 8.7 Bar = 1 cm.

## Questions

1. Describe any abnormalities.
2. Provide a diagnosis.
3. How would you link these lesions to this dog's death?

# HAEM8

## Topics

Practical technique

Lesion recognition

Common artefacts and pitfalls

## History

An adult, female domestic shorthair cat presented for necropsy. It had been a rescue cat which had presented with anorexia, weight loss and chronic anaemia.

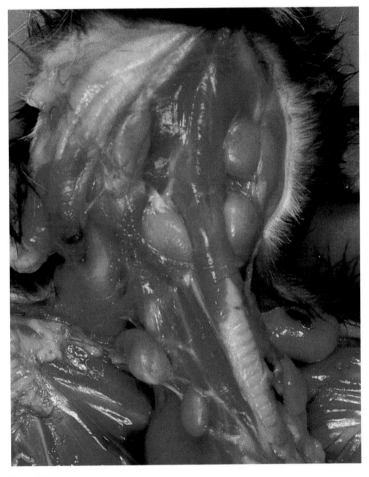

Fig. 8.8

## Questions

1. Describe any abnormalities.
2. Provide a diagnosis.
3. How might you try to clarify the most likely diagnosis at the time of necropsy, i.e. prior to pursuing any histopathology?

# HAEM9

## Topics

**Lesion recognition**

**Pathogenesis**

## History

A 3Y old, female neutered Ragdoll cat presented with a history of lethargy, inappetance, vomiting blood, and altered faeces (Fig. 8.9). On clinical examination, the mucous membranes were paler than normal. Haematology confirmed mild neutropaenia and severe thrombocytopaenia. Additional testing showed that the cat was positive for feline immunode-ficiency virus (FIV). Despite supportive therapy, the cat deteriorated suddenly and died. The most significant necropsy findings are highlighted in Figs 8.10–8.12.

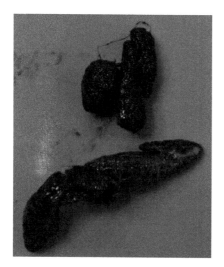

Fig. 8.9

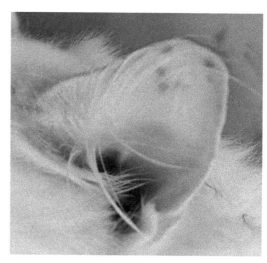

Fig. 8.10

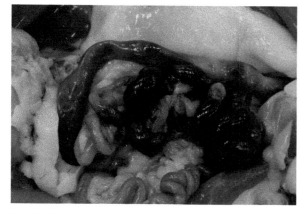

Fig. 8.11

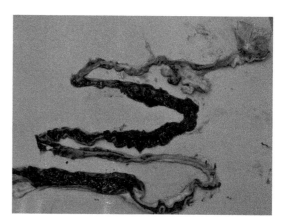

Fig. 8.12

## Questions

1. Describe any abnormalities in Figs 8.9–8.12.
2. Provide a diagnosis.
3. Provide some possible causes of thrombocytopaenia in cats and dogs and explain how this leads to the changes in this case.

# HAEM1 answers

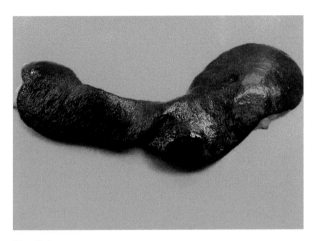

Fig. 8.1

## 1. Describe any abnormalities

In the body of the spleen, slightly elevating the parietal surface, there is a well-demarcated, soft (probably!), dark purple/red, wedge-shaped lesion, measuring approximately 3 × 2 cm.

## 2. Provide a diagnosis

Focal acute splenic infarct.

> In addition to its well-demarcated border, a key feature of this lesion is that it is only slightly raised – it is not forming a nodule as such.

## 3. Provide some potential underlying causes for this lesion and suggest how you might link this lesion to the icterus

Regardless of location, an infarct is defined as an area of necrosis following blockage of a supplying blood vessel. Vessel obstruction is usually due to formation of a fibrin thrombus (or thromboembolus, when a thrombus forms, travels to another part of the vasculature and becomes lodged there), otherwise known as thrombosis (or thromboembolism). Virchow's triad dictates that thrombosis may be caused by (1) stasis of blood flow (2) changes in blood coagulability (3) and/or vessel wall damage. Within each

of these three categories there are many potential causes but common ones include sepsis, disseminated intravascular coagulopathy, hypercorticism, underlying neoplasia, protein-losing nephropathy and vasculitis.[1]

Icterus may have a pre-hepatic, hepatic or post-hepatic origin. The history in this case tends to support pre-hepatic icterus, which is usually due to haemolysis. Haemolysis may be immune mediated or non-immune mediated. Immune-mediated haemolytic anaemia (IMHA) is classed as primary (generally idiopathic) or secondary. Cocker spaniels are predisposed to primary IMHA (another clue in this example) but they are not the only predisposed breed; others include Poodles, Irish setters and English springer spaniels.[2] IMHA is often complicated by an inflammatory leukocytosis and a coagulopathy, leading to thrombosis and providing a link to the infarct in this case. The exact mechanism of IMHA associated thrombosis is not crystal clear, mainly because it is complex and multifactorial. For instance, cell membranes from ruptured erythrocytes are pro-coagulant, as is the prolonged steroid therapy that often underpins treatment of these cases. Haemolysis-induced hypoxia often leads to liver necrosis, which may at least partially explain the liver's role in generating thrombi.[2]

In the spleen it is important to be aware that there can be focal areas of dark red discolouration due to pooling of blood at either pole, or elsewhere if there is incomplete contraction. If unsure whether the change you see is an infarct or just a focal area of congestion, always take a sample for histology.

## References

1  Mosier, D. A. (2017). Vascular disorders and thrombosis. In J. F. Zachary (Ed.) *Pathologic basis of veterinary disease* (6th ed). Elsevier. https://doi.org/10.1016/B978-0-323-35775-3.00002-3

2  Carr, A. P., Panciera, D. L., & Kidd, L. (2002). Prognostic factors for mortality and thromboembolism in canine immune-mediated hemolytic anemia: A retrospective study of 72 dogs. *Journal of Veterinary Internal Medicine*, 16(5), 504–509. https://doi.org/10.1111/j.1939-1676.2002.tb02378.x

# HAEM2 answers

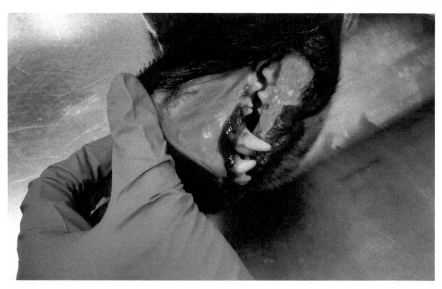

Fig. 8.2

## 1.   Describe any abnormalities
The oral mucosa is diffusely bright yellow/orange.

## 2.   Provide a diagnosis
Icterus (or jaundice). Fig. 8.2a below illustrates the extent of this lesion.

> Note: This is really a morphological diagnosis, which is completely acceptable for the purposes of these cases.

## 3.   Outline the main potential causes of this condition, taking into considering any health and safety implications
Regardless of cause, icterus is defined as hyperbilirubinaemia, i.e. too much circulating bilirubin. It is normal to have small amounts of bilirubin in circulation, since it is a direct consequence of erythrocyte breakdown. Once erythrocytes have expired, they are digested by macrophages and their haemoglobin (Hb) is broken down. Hb comprises haem, iron and amino acids. The amino acids are recycled, the iron removed and the haem converted to biliverdin, then bilirubin.

Pre-hepatic icterus is due to haemolysis, during which there is overwhelming release and breakdown of Hb and, consequently, too much circulating bilirubin. The amount of bilirubin exceeds the capacity of the liver to metabolise it. Haemolytic anaemia is most commonly immune-mediated in veterinary species. It occurs in both dogs and cats but is more common in the dog. Antibodies bind to the cell membrane of red blood cells, in turn interacting with complement, which ultimately leads to haemolysis. Immune-mediated haemolytic anaemia (IMHA) may be primary – otherwise known as idiopathic – or secondary. In primary IMHA, a cause is not identified but secondary IMHA is usually due to another underlying disease process which may be infectious, neoplastic or chemical (e.g. therapeutic agents, vaccines or toxins). Diagnostic steps include a complete blood count and blood smear evaluation specifically for spherocytes (this is only appropriate for dogs, not cats); a positive saline agglutination test; and detection of antibodies directed against red blood cells (flow cytometry and direct Coomb's test).[1]

Hepatic icterus arises when diseased hepatocytes cannot maintain the normal pace of bilirubin uptake or bile production and/or secretion. Normally, bilirubin is initially unconjugated and reaches the liver in the bloodstream attached to albumin. Hepatocytes attach (conjugate) bilirubin to glucuronic acid, so that the bilirubin becomes water soluble. The conjugated bilirubin is excreted in bile with water, bile acids and cholesterol. If uptake and conjugation of bilirubin by hepatocytes cannot take place due to reduced hepatocellular function, or if they cannot synthesise bile, then plasma bilirubin levels will increase. The potential causes of hepatic icterus are thus myriad, as there are many potential causes of hepatocellular injury.

Post-hepatic icterus results from blockage of the biliary tree, particularly the main bile duct.

The main health and safety implication to be aware of in cases of icterus is underlying leptospirosis which is, of course, potentially zoonotic. Dogs are susceptible to various serovars (main ones are *L. canicola,*

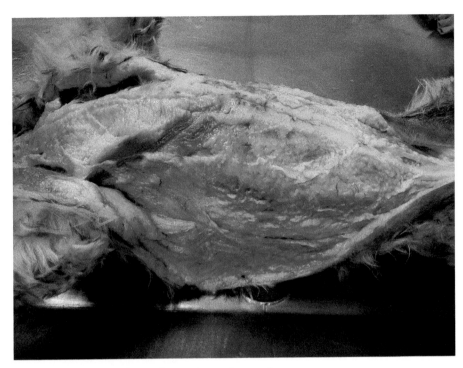

Fig. 8.2a  Orange/yellow subcutaneous fat, canine.

*L. icterohaemorrhagiae, L. pomona,* and *L. grippotyphosa*). Vaccination history is therefore pertinent in such instances.

Severe icterus is often pre-hepatic (i.e. haemolytic), as in this dog. This particular breed is predisposed to immune-mediated haemolytic anaemia, which was the diagnosis in this case. In addition to bright yellow to orange subcutaneous fat, other mucosal surfaces, internal fat and sclera are usually also similarly discoloured and were in this case.

## Reference

1  Garden, O. A., Kidd, L., Mexas, A. M., Chang, Y. M., Jeffery, U., Blois, S. L., Fogle, J. E., MacNeill, A. L., Lubas, G., Birkenheuer, A., Buoncompagni, S., Dandrieux, J. R. S., Di Loria, A., Fellman, C. L., Glanemann, B., Goggs, R., Granick, J. L., LeVine, D. N., Sharp, C. R., . . . Szladovits, B. (2019). ACVIM consensus statement on the diagnosis of immune-mediated hemolytic anemia in dogs and cats. *Journal of Veterinary Internal Medicine,* 33(2), 313–334. https://doi.org/10.1111/jvim.15441

# HAEM3 answers

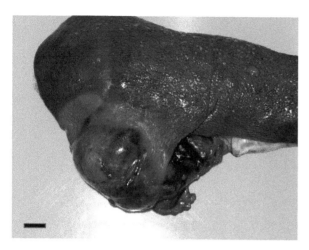

Fig. 8.3

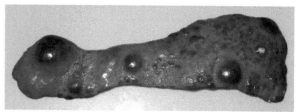

Fig. 8.3a Multifocal nodular lymphoid hyperplasia, canine spleen. Canine spleen, parietal surface: There are multiple (>10), raised, well-demarcated, dark red, smooth, spherical nodules scattered throughout the spleen, ranging in diameter up to ~ 2 cm. One nodule is mostly pale yellow and, for this reason, we can probably be a little more confident that this reflects nodular hyperplasia.

## 1. Describe any abnormalities

At one pole of the spleen there is a focal, raised, smooth, ovoid mass that is mottled pink, tan and dark red. It is soft, measures approximately 3 × 4 cm and is partially circumscribed by a pale pink/tan rim measuring up to 1 cm thick. There is also a 5 mm diameter, raised, pink nodule on the parietal surface of the spleen, surrounded by myriad, shiny, smooth, grey, pinpoint plaques.

## 2. Provide a diagnosis

The red mass could be splenic nodular hyperplasia, a haematoma or haemangiosarcoma. We cannot be definitive without histopathology.

The 5 mm pink nodule may be a small nodule of hyperplasia or capsular fibrosis.

The grey pinpoint lesions are small foci of capsular fibrosis (probably a precursor to siderofibrotic plaque formation).

## 3. What is the clinical significance of any lesion(s) identified?

Haematomas and nodular hyperplasia are benign and non-neoplastic. They often occur together in the same lesion. If there is any haematoma component, then there is the risk of rupture and acute haemorrhage (which could be fatal in severe cases) or simply just chronic low-grade haemorrhage leading to anaemia. Splenic haemangiosarcoma is, of course, a malignant neoplasm of endothelial (or possibly marrow progenitor) cell origin. It carries a high risk of widespread metastasis and can also rupture and haemorrhage, leading to haemoabdomen and sudden death. It can be very difficult to distinguish these grossly. Fig. 8.3a depicts how nodular lymphoid hyperplasia can be multifocal. However, so too can haemangiosarcoma and it would be a brave clinician

or pathologist who would rule out haemangiosarcoma without histopathology. Capsular fibrosis is incidental, as is siderofibrotic plaque formation. Such lesions are often considered age related and may be secondary to some sort of trauma or local irritation.

> ### TIP
> When sampling this type of very haemorrhagic nodule (in any organ but particularly the spleen), always sample the transition with surrounding more solid tissue, as well as the lesion, as this is where neoplastic cells are most likely to appreciable. See Fig. 8.3b for suggested approach.
>
> A better alternative is to send the entire spleen to your pathologist as this minimises the risk of missing something important and also allows further bites at the cherry – so to speak – as usually the fixed submitted organ will be retained for a short period of time, allowing later review as necessary.
>
>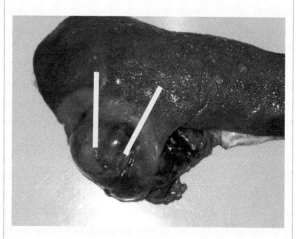
>
> Fig. 8.3b Canine spleen. Yellow lines denote best plane of section for sampling.

# HAEM4 answers

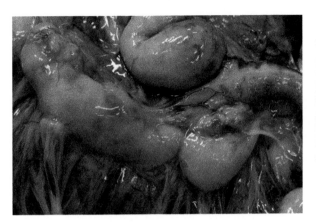

Fig. 8.4

### 1. Describe any abnormalities

Multiple intra-abdominal lymph nodes (mesenteric) are markedly enlarged and diffusely pale fawn with a smooth, rounded surface. The intestine dorsal to the enlarged nodes is the ileocaecocolic junction.

### 2. Provide a diagnosis

Lymphoma – mesenteric lymph nodes.

### 3. Outline some differential diagnoses

In the dog, lymphoma is the most likely diagnosis for this type of presentation. On cut section of a lymph node in an established case, the normal nodal architecture is replaced by homogeneous, white to off-white tissue that characteristically bulges on cut section, usually because there is little supporting stroma (Fig. 8.4a). Other round cell tumours are potential differentials, such as a mast cell tumour or a large granular lymphoma/leukaemia. Histiocytic sarcoma can also present in a similar way but does not usually bulge in the way that lymphoma does. Impression smears at time of necropsy will often provide a good indication of most likely diagnosis (staining with Giemsa is best but Diff-Quik of a well-preserved specimen will often suffice).

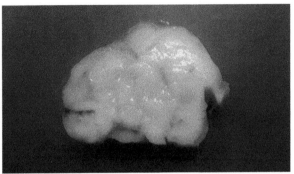

Fig. 8.4a Canine lymph node with lymphoma.

### Comment

Lymphoma is really a misnomer since the suffix '-oma' implies that it is benign. Though now considered an old-fashioned term, lymphosarcoma is more accurate since the suffix '-sarcoma' denotes malignancy of mesenchymal origin, and lymphoma is always malignant. The presentation in this case correlates best with multicentric lymphoma, which will often manifest as peripheral lymphadenopathy, progressing to involve the liver, spleen and eventually other organs, including the bone marrow. This is the most common form of lymphoma in the dog and it is more commonly of B cell origin. More indolent forms may only affect one or two lymph nodes and are more slowly progressive; they are less common, however. Other manifestations of canine lymphoma are gastrointestinal, cutaneous, thymic and central nervous system.

### Reference

1   Zandvliet, M. (2016). Canine lymphoma: A review. *Veterinary Quarterly*, *36*, 76–104. https://doi.org/10.1080/01652176.2016.1152633

# HAEM5 answers

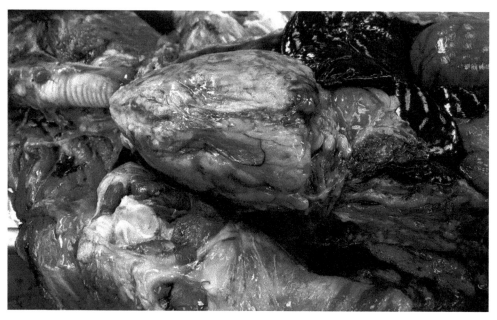

Fig. 8.5

## 1.   Describe any abnormalities

A pale yellow/cream-coloured mass fills the cranial thoracic cavity, obscuring much of the heart and both lungs. The liver lies between the stomach (top right of image) and the thoracic mass. It is somewhat darker than normal.

## 2.   Provide a diagnosis

Thymoma or thymic lymphoma are the two most likely differentials for this type of solid mass occupying much of the cranial mediastinum.

## 3.

### a)   Name at least TWO conditions or other lesions associated with your diagnosis

Associated with thymoma: Megaoesophagus; myasthenia gravis; polymyositis/myositis; rarely, paraneoplastic conditions such as hypercalcaemia, erythema multiforme or myocarditis.[1,2]

Associated with thymic lymphoma: Pleural effusion; hypercalcaemia (due to humoral hypercalcaemia of malignancy) or vena cava syndrome.[3,4]

### b)   List some other differentials for a mass within the cranial thoracic cavity

Other differentials include a thyroid carcinoma, especially arising from ectopic thyroid tissue, metastatic carcinoma, or a heart base tumour (e.g. aortic body tumour).[1]

Granulomatous inflammation can sometimes present as a solid, space-occupying lesion and can quite easily mimic a neoplastic process. Mesothelioma usually appears less localised and solid. It is usually more dispersed/multifocal and florid with formation of fronds. Always make sure that the mass is not continuous with the ribs. Though more unusual, it would introduce differentials such as a chondrosarcoma.

> Note: The German Shepherd Dog is predisposed to thymoma.[1]

## References

1   Robat, C. S., Cesario, L., Gaeta, R., Miller, M., Schrempp, D., & Chun, R. (2013). Clinical features, treatment options, and outcome in dogs with thymoma: 116 cases (1999–2010). *Journal of the American Veterinary Medical Association*, 243(10), 1448–1454. https://doi.org/10.2460/javma.243.10.1448

2   Aronsohn, M. (1985). Canine thymoma. *Veterinary Clinics of North America. Small Animal Practice*, 15(4), 755–767. https://doi.org/10.1016/s0195-5616(85)50034-0

3   Zandvliet, M. (2016). Canine lymphoma: A review. *Veterinary Quarterly*. Web of Science, 36(2), 76–104. https://doi.org/10.1080/01652176.2016.1152633

4   Fan, T. M. (2019). Canine lymphoma. MSD Veterinary Manual. msdvetmanual.com

# HAEM6 answers

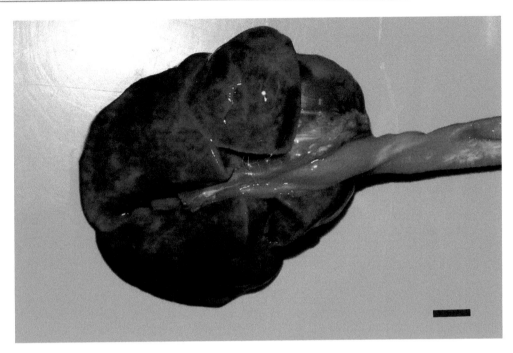

Fig. 8.6 **Bar = 1 cm.**

## 1.  Describe any abnormalities

There is no thymus, which should be present in an animal of this age. The lungs are also diffusely mottled dark red which may be a postmortem artefact, although concomitant mild interstitial pneumonia is a reasonable differential.

## 2.  Provide a diagnosis

Severe thymic atrophy.

## 3.  Based on the history, outline some differential diagnoses and the possible pathogenesis of this lesion

Potential differentials for prolonged vomiting and diarrhoea in a puppy include parvovirus infection (high on the list); severe endoparasitism (e.g. *Toxocara canis;* coccidiosis); dietary indiscretion; and intestinal obstruction (e.g. foreign body; intussusception). Potential causes in older dogs include neoplasia, chronic enteropathy (e.g. inflammatory bowel disease) and organ failure, but are much less likely in such a young dog. Other infections are a possible consideration, although lower down the differential list (e.g. *Salmonella*). While some other infectious diseases may cause vomiting and diarrhoea, additional clinical signs may be expected too (e.g. canine distemper may also be associated with conjunctivitis, rhinitis, pneumonia, etc).

Thymic atrophy is usually caused by either viral infection (especially canine parvovirus and canine distemper virus) or severe stress. However, it may also occur with malnutrition/nutritional deficiencies, toxin exposure or iatrogenically due to drug therapy.[1] The thymus eventually disappears with age, but this is known as involution, not atrophy.

The main differential in this case is thymic hypoplasia. With thymic atrophy, there would have been a normal thymus at birth, but rapid depletion of lymphocytes due to infection, stress etc. would lead to loss of thymic tissue. In contrast, a hypoplastic thymus never grows fully in the first place. It can be difficult to distinguish between the two, but atrophy is much more likely to be the cause, particularly where there is, or has been, underlying illness.

> **TIP**
>
> This is a very good example of a case where the lesion is a missing organ – you need to remember to look for it in order to identify the abnormality. Similar examples include unilateral renal aplasia, lack of a spleen (perhaps due to previous surgery), cerebellar hypoplasia, and situs inversus (rare).

## Reference

1  Valli, V. E. O., Kiupel, M., & Bienzle, D. (2016). Haematopoietic system. In M. G. Maxie (Ed.), *Jubb, Kennedy and Palmer's pathology of domestic animals* (6th ed), Vol. 3. Elsevier. https://doi.org/10.1016/B978-0-7020-5319-1.00013-X

# HAEM7 answers

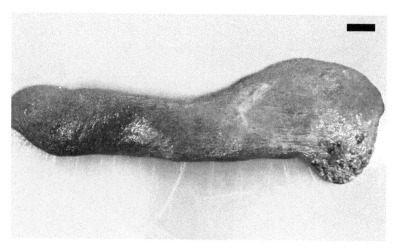

Fig. 8.7 Bar = 1 cm.

## 1.   Describe any abnormalities

This is the spleen. On the capsular surface of the head of the spleen there are multifocal to coalescing raised, smooth, red to golden, circular lesions and crust-like plaques that range in size up to ~3 mm. There is also a flat, linear, ill-defined grey area at the junction between the head and body of the spleen. See a higher magnification in Fig. 8.7a.

## 2.   Provide a diagnosis

(a)   Moderate multifocal to coalescing capsular siderofibrosis (siderofibrotic plaque formation).

(b)   Focal capsular fibrosis.

## 3.   How would you link these lesions to this dog's death?

They are not linked. Both lesions are incidental and pre-existing. Siderofibrotic plaques (also known as Gamna-Gandy bodies) are believed to be due to previous low-grade trauma and are broadly understood to be age related in the dog. Similarly, capsular fibrosis is likely due to previous low-grade irritation or trauma on the capsular surface. Histologically, siderofibrotic plaques correspond to areas of mineralisation, fibrosis, haemosiderosis and haematoidin deposition. The haemosiderin and haematoidin confer the distinct golden appearance grossly. It is important to recognise this as a clinically insignificant lesion during, for example, exploratory laparotomy – it is no reason to remove the spleen if it is otherwise normal.

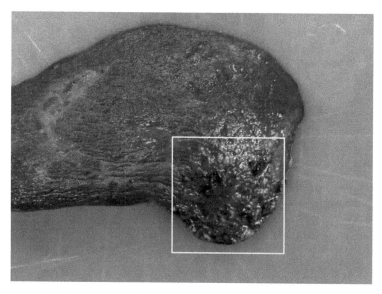

Fig. 8.7a Higher magnification of canine splenic lesion in Fig. 8.11.

# HAEM8 answers

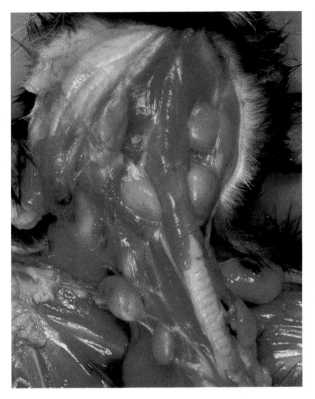

Fig. 8.8

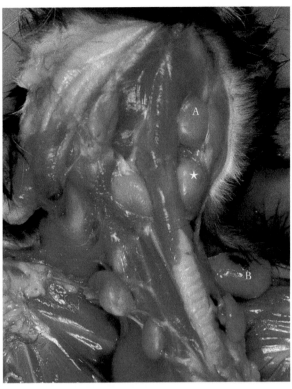

Fig. 8.8a **Feline ventral neck. A: Left mandibular lymph node. B: Left prescapular lymph node. \* Left submandibular salivary gland.**

## 1.   Describe any abnormalities

The mandibular and prescapular lymph nodes are all bilaterally markedly enlarged and pale tan with rounded borders. There is a red blood clot on the surface of the left prescapular lymph node. Two lymph nodes caudal to the prescapular lymph nodes are likely cervical but are not as markedly enlarged. See annotated version in 8.8a.

## 2.   Provide a diagnosis

Lymphoma is most likely, given the number of nodes affected. The main differentials are reactive lymphoid hyperplasia and, less likely, lymphadenitis.

## 3.   How might you try to clarify the most likely diagnosis at the time of necropsy, i.e. prior to pursuing any histopathology?

a)   Section the lymph node. In a node with established lymphoma, the normal nodal structure will be replaced by solid, pale tan to white tissue which will likely bulge a little towards you as the neoplastic lymphocytes have very little supportive stroma to 'hold them in place'. In a reactive lymph node there will still be appreciable cortical and medullary architecture. A reactive node contains hyperplastic cortex with enlarged lymphoid follicles and germinal centres so the outer cortex will be whiter and will bulge a little more compared to the medulla, which will usually be pale

tan. The medulla may be red if there is drainage of blood through the node.

b)   Make some impression smears of the lymph node parenchyma. Cut the node and blot the cut surface to get rid of excess liquid. Be very gentle. Lymphocytes are fragile and rupture easily. Dab gently against the slide – if the cut surface is small you can dab three or four times in a row on the same slide. If you have access to a Giemsa based stain, then use this as it offers better contrast and nuclear detail, but Diff-Quik is fine if it is all you have. If the animal has been dead for some time, cytology is less useful. In a normal lymph node, small lymphocytes will predominate (~90% of lymphocytes) though there will be a few medium sized and large lymphocytes, as well as a few plasma cells and macrophages. In lymphoma, you should see a monomorphous population of lymphocytes, often medium sized to large† depending on the type of lymphoma present.

† Small lymphocyte nuclei are 1–1.5× the diameter of an RBC in cytological preparations. Medium sized lymphocyte nuclei are 2–2.5× the diameter of an RBC. Large lymphocyte nuclei are >3× the diameter of an RBC.

See Case URIN3 for a good example of a cytological smear from a case of feline lymphoma.

c)   Evaluation of other organs will also be helpful in the necropsy situation – spleen, liver, kidneys and GI tract are often also involved in feline lymphoma[1] – in fact, the multicentric presentation observed frequently in dogs is much less common in cats. Look for features such as diffuse splenomegaly, hepatomegaly, renomegaly or nodular tan lesions in these organs.

---

TIP

Evaluation of the cut surface is often very helpful. It can also be used to distinguish lymph node from salivary gland – e.g. the submandibular salivary gland in Fig. 8.8a above would have much more of an even lobular pattern throughout, a pattern that would be absent from a lymph node.

Cut section also helps distinguish adrenal or thyroid glands from regional lymph nodes and pancreas from surrounding fat.

So … do not forget the cut surface.

---

## Reference

1   Mason, S., & Pittaway, C. (2022). Feline lymphoma: Diagnosis, staging and clinical presentations. *In Practice*, 44(1) (January/February), 4–20. https://doi.org/10.1002/inpr.163

# HAEM9 answers

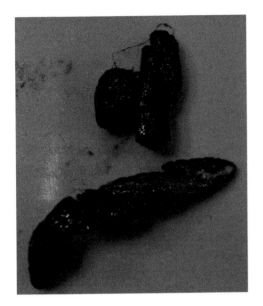

Fig. 8.9

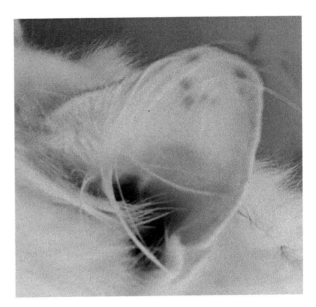

Fig. 8.10

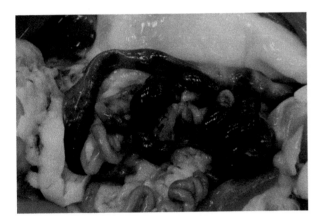

Fig. 8.11

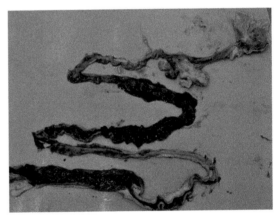

Fig. 8.12

## 1. Describe any abnormalities in Figs 8.9–8.12

Fig. 8.9: The faeces are darker than normal (virtually black), consistent with melena.

Fig 8.10: There are multifocal, small (approximately 1–2 mm) red foci over the inner aspect of the left pinna (petechiae).

Fig 8.11 and 8.12: There is segmental swelling and dark red discolouration of the small intestine with a large amount of luminal haemorrhage and melena evident once the tract is opened. A hair ball is also present in the stomach.

## 2. Provide a diagnosis

Thrombocytopaenia with cutaneous petechial haemorrhage and severe, subacute intra-intestinal haemorrhage.

## 3. Provide some possible causes of thrombocytopaenia in cats and dogs and explain how this leads to the changes in this case

Thrombocytopaenia may be due to:

a. decreased production of platelets e.g. following bone marrow damage/destruction by infectious agents e.g. canine/feline parvovirus, FeLV, FIV, anaplasma, mycoplasma etc; neoplasia (e.g. leukaemia or metastatic spread to bone marrow); drug therapy (e.g. chemotherapeutic drugs, oestrogen, etc.); or myelofibrosis (which may occur secondary to bone marrow damage).

b. increased destruction or consumption of platelets e.g. primary immune-mediated thrombocytopaenia (especially dogs); disseminated intravascular coagulopathy, etc.

c. thrombopathias, e.g. inherited platelet dysfunction disorders.[1,2]

---

**TIP**

Surface (mucosal, epidermal, serosal etc) haemorrhage is usually classified based on the size of the areas of haemorrhage as follows:

- Petechiae are smallest, measuring 1–2 mm. They are generally due to increased blood pressure or disorders of primary haemostasis, such as thrombocytopaenia.
- Purpura usually measure ≥3 mm.
- Ecchymoses measure 1–3 cm.
- Anything larger is classed as 'suffusive'.[2]

---

Thrombocytopaenia results in failure of primary haemostasis (i.e. the formation of the platelet plug) and animals may present with petechial and ecchymotic haemorrhages over the skin and mucosal surfaces (as in this case)[3]. Severe spontaneous haemorrhage may occur following minor trauma (or diagnostic procedures). In this case, there was severe, fatal, gastrointestinal haemorrhage secondary to thrombocytopaenia due to FIV infection, which resulted in the sudden demise of the cat.

## References

1   Ellis, J., Bell, R., Barnes, D. C., & Miller, R. (2018). Prevalence and disease associations in feline thrombocytopenia: A retrospective study of 194 cases. *Journal of Small Animal Practice,* *59*(9), 531–538. https://doi.org/10.1111/jsap.12814

2   Mosier, D. A. (2017). Vascular disorders and thrombosis. In J. F. Zachary (Ed.) *Pathologic basis of veterinary disease* (6th ed). Elsevier. https://doi.org/10.1016/B978-0-323-35775-3.00002-3

3   Kumar, A. K. Abbas & J. C. Aster (2021). Robbins & Cotran pathologic basis of disease (10th ed). Elsevier.

# Reproductive cases

**9**

# REPRO1

## Topics

Practical technique

Lesion recognition

Prioritisation of findings

## History

This was one of several lesions found in a 10Y old, male Collie cross that had been euthanised on humane grounds, due to metastatic carcinoma.

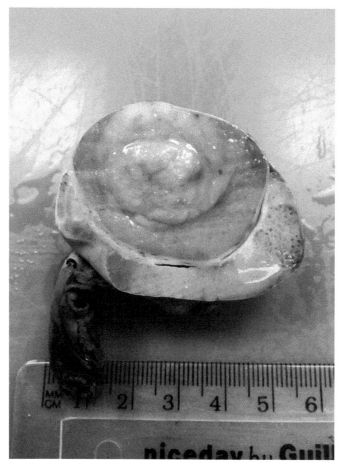

Fig. 9.1

## Questions

1. Describe any abnormalities.
2. Provide a diagnosis.
3. How significant was this likely to have been in terms of this dog's metastatic disease and clinical outcome?

# REPRO2

## Topics

Lesion recognition

Integration of pathological findings with clinical aspects

Pathogenesis

## History

Figs 9.2 and 9.3 are necropsy findings in a 9Y old, male mixed-breed dog. Fig. 9.2 illustrates a cryptorchid testis (see Fig. 9.4 for in situ image).

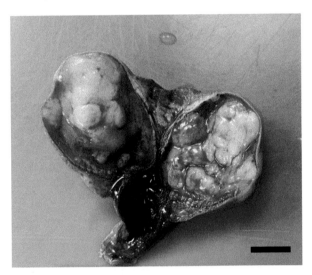

Fig. 9.2 **Bar = 1 cm.**

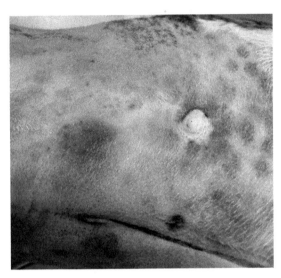

Fig. 9.3

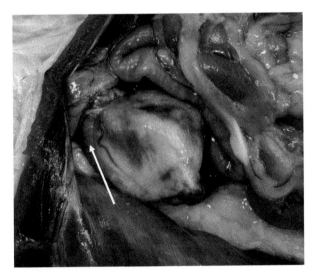

Fig. 9.4 Cryptorchid testis (white arrow points to epididymis).

## Questions

1. Describe any abnormalities in Figs 9.2 and 9.3.
2. Provide a diagnosis.
3. What is the likely behaviour of this lesion in the live animal? Link this with the features in Fig. 9.3.

# REPRO3

## Topics

**Lesion recognition**

**Pathogenesis**

## History

The image in Fig. 9.5 shows an apparently incidental necropsy finding in a 7Y old, intact female Scottish Terrier, which had been euthanised for unrelated reasons.

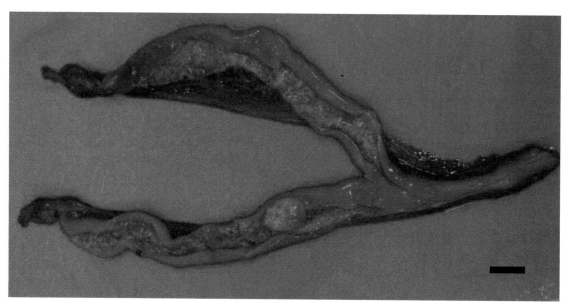

Fig. 9.5  **Bar = 1 cm.**

## Questions

1. Describe any abnormalities.
2. Provide a diagnosis.
3. Briefly outline how progesterone and oestrogen influence the development of this lesion.

# REPRO4

## Topic

**Lesion recognition**

## History

Fig. 9.6 shows an image of an incidental necropsy finding from a 10Y old, male Labrador crossbreed dog.

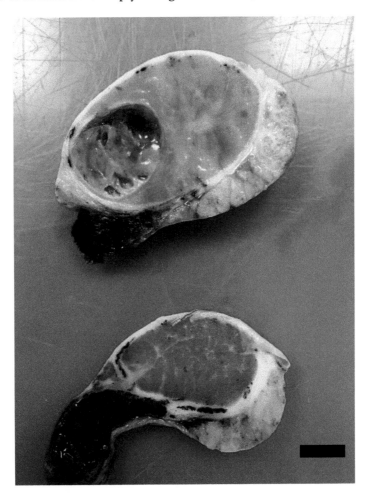

Fig. 9.6  Bar = 1 cm.

## Questions

1. Describe any abnormalities.
2. Provide a diagnosis.
3. Which gross features justify your diagnosis?

# REPRO5

## Topics

**Lesion recognition**

**Pathogenesis**

**Integration of pathological findings with clinical aspects**

## History

A 6Y old, female intact Golden Retriever presented with a history of anorexia, vomiting, abdominal discomfort, polyuria and polydipsia and was diagnosed with a closed pyometra (no vaginal discharge present). The Retriever underwent ovariohysterectomy but there was evidence of peritonitis at the time of surgery. The dog did not recover well despite supportive therapy and subsequently was submitted for necropsy along with the surgically removed uterus, which had been placed in formalin at time of surgery. The main necropsy findings were a moderate pleural effusion and petechial haemorrhage on multiple lymph nodes and on the peritoneal surface.

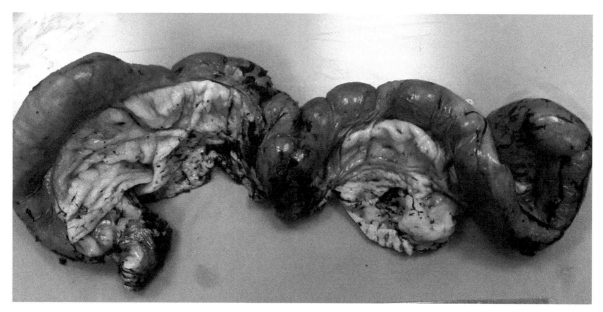

Fig. 9.7

## Questions

1. Describe any abnormalities.
2. Provide a diagnosis.
3. Outline the pathogenesis of this condition and most likely reasons for this dog's (a) polyuria and (b) death.

# REPRO6

## Topic covered

**Lesion recognition**

## History

Fig. 9.8 illustrates an incidental necropsy finding in a young, male intact Cocker Spaniel found dead by its owners one morning.

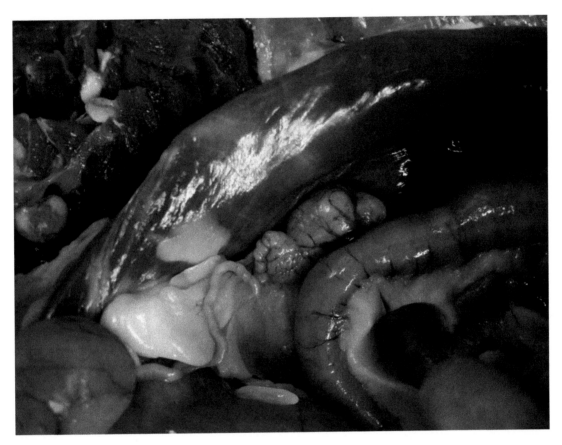

Fig. 9.8

## Questions

1. Describe any abnormalities.
2. Provide a diagnosis.
3. This is now classified as a disorder of sexual development (DSD). Briefly outline:
   a.  The cause of this condition.
   b.  Potential consequences.

# REPRO7

## Topics

**Lesion recognition**

**Pathogenesis**

## History

A 10Y old, male intact Airedale Terrier presented in abdominal pain, with haematuria and dysuria. There was marked discomfort on abdominal palpation, with detection of a mass caudal to the urinary bladder, further confirmed on abdominal ultrasound. After a brief period of treatment, the dog stopped eating, developing persistent vomiting with melaena so the owners made the decision to euthanise. Fig. 9.9 shows the mass.

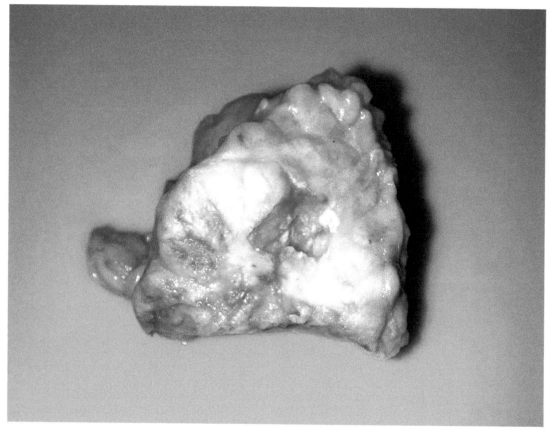

Fig. 9.9

## Questions

1. Describe any abnormalities.
2. Provide a diagnosis.
3. How would you expect this lesion to behave and how would you distinguish it from benign prostatic hyperplasia?

# REPRO8

## Topics

Lesion recognition

Generation of pathological differential diagnoses lists

## History

The image in Fig. 9.10 is the main necropsy finding in a 10Y old, male entire Boxer dog with a history of chronic heart failure due to dilated cardiomyopathy and chronic degenerative joint disease. The dog presented with a swollen, painful and warm scrotal area and a history of anorexia and stilted gait. The dog was euthanised at the owner's request due to concerns over the risks of surgery.

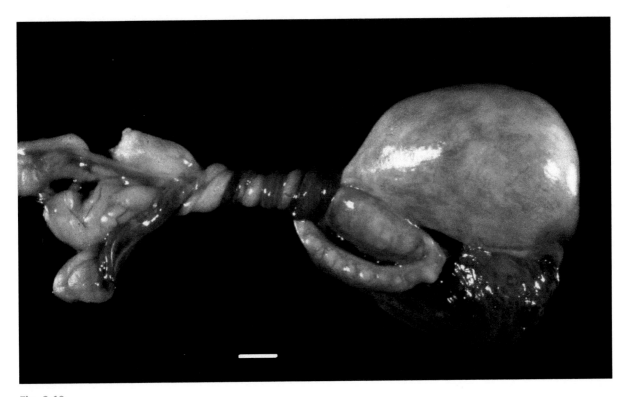

Fig. 9.10

## Questions

1. Describe any abnormalities.
2. Provide a diagnosis.
3. Outline three other potential causes of scrotal swelling in the dog.

# REPRO1 answers

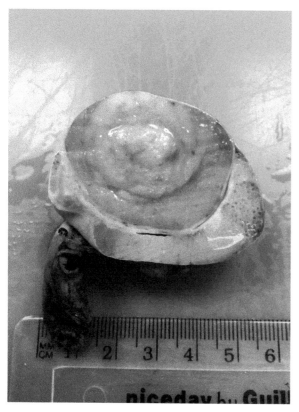

Fig. 9.1

This example is pink-tinged because it is not completely fixed. Even when fresh they are often completely white but they may have areas of necrosis or haemorrhage within (compare with a more fully fixed seminoma in Fig. 9.1a). They have a homogeneous, soft texture and tend to bulge on cut section, mainly because they do not have much supportive stroma. In that respect they mimic lymphoma a little.

> **TIP**
>
> Always 'bread loaf' (that is, serially section at ~3–4 mm intervals) both testes during a necropsy to ensure you do not miss a lesion. Testicular neoplasms are common in older dogs. If submitting testes as a biopsy from a live dog, always include the spermatic cord, notably the pampiniform plexus, so that the pathologist can examine these areas. Although malignant testicular tumours are not common, malignant cells can invade and infiltrate along the vessels to the peritoneal cavity, as well as tissues around the testis (so submit testis, epididymis and pampiniform plexus en bloc).

### 1.  Describe any abnormalities

This is testis, epididymis and pampiniform plexus. The testis contains a well-demarcated, soft, pale pink/white, bulging mass that measures 2.75 cm diameter and is mildly compressive.

### 2.  Provide a diagnosis

Testicular seminoma.

### 3.  How significant was this likely to have been in terms of this dog's metastatic disease and clinical outcome?

Probably not significant at all. Seminomas originate from the germ cells in the seminiferous tubules and generally do not metastasise, although a small percentage can. They do not fall into the category of carcinoma so were not directly related to the metastatic carcinoma in this dog. This was most likely an incidental additional finding in this case.

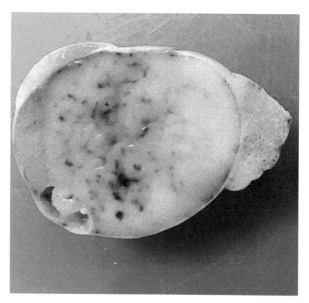

Fig. 9.1a **Testicular seminoma, canine.**

# REPRO2 answers

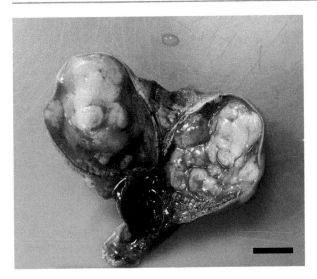

Fig. 9.2 Bar = 1 cm.

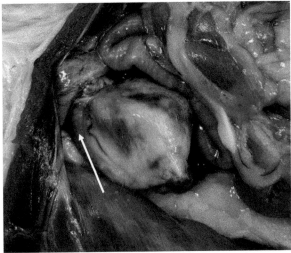

Fig. 9.4 Cryptorchid testis (white arrow points to epididymis).

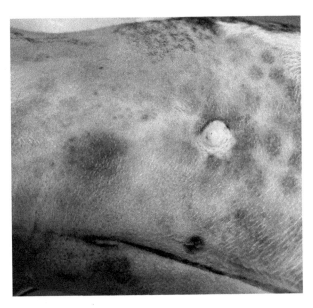

Fig. 9.3

## 1.  Describe any abnormalities in Figs 9.2 and 9.3.

Fig 9.2: There is no normal testicular tissue remaining (almost no longer recognisable). Most of the normal architecture is replaced by a multilobulated, well-demarcated, white, slightly bulging mass that measures approximately 3 cm × 2.5 cm × 1 cm.

Fig 9.3: There is thinning of the hair coat along the ventrum, and multiple ill-defined red foci on the skin, ranging from pinpoint to approximately 2 cm diameter (hyperaemia and/or petechial to ecchymotic haemorrhage).

## 2.  Provide a diagnosis

This is a sustentacular (Sertoli) cell tumour, arising from supportive sustentacular cells of the seminiferous tubules. Cryptorchid testes are predisposed to neoplasia but this tumour can arise in an otherwise normal testis.

Compare this example with REPRO1. Even though it is an image, you can still appreciate that this tumour has a more striated surface (see Fig. 9.4a) which suggests it is firmer. That is because these tumours have a more abundant supportive stroma compared to seminomas so it is a helpful distinguishing feature grossly. The areas of haemorrhage may be just that. However, another consideration is a concomitant interstitial (Leydig) cell tumour, since this type of neoplasm often has cystic areas filled with blood. It is also common to see more than one tumour type in the same testis concurrently.

## 3.  What is the likely behaviour of this lesion in the live animal? Link this with the features in Fig. 9.3.

These tumours are usually benign, as are most canine testicular tumours; only a small percentage are malignant but malignant forms can rarely metastasise to regional lymph nodes and internal organs.[1] It is well established that dogs with this type of tumour may develop feminisation syndrome, characterised by gynaecomastia, attractiveness to other males, pendulous prepuce, lethargy, atrophy of the other testis, alopecia, squamous metaplasia of the prostate gland and, most importantly, bone marrow suppression,

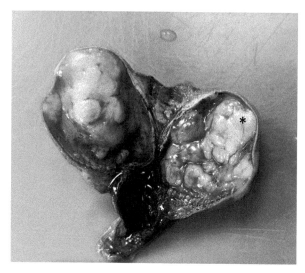

Fig. 9.4a Black asterisk denotes slightly striated area.

which may lead to anaemia, thrombocytopaenia and leukopaenia.[1,2] Feminisation occurs in approximately 25%

of affected dogs. Not all cases are associated with elevated oestrogen, however, and the exact mechanism is unclear (secretion of oestrogen by the tumour; conversion of male hormones to oestrogen, general sex hormonal imbalance may all be involved). Fig. 9.3 depicts hair thinning but also has areas of hyperaemia and possible haemorrhage. Hyperaemia is recognised in conjunction with alopecia in feminisation syndrome, though the smaller foci of haemorrhage (petechiae) could be secondary to thrombocytopaenia.

## References

1 Foster, R. A. (2012). Common lesions in the male reproductive tract of cats and dogs. *Veterinary Clinics of North America. Small Animal Practice*, *42*(3), 527–545. https://doi.org/10.1016/j.cvsm.2012.01.007

2 Foster, R. A. (2016). Male genital system. In In M. G. Maxie (Ed.), *Jubb, Kennedy and Palmer's pathology of domestic animals* (6th ed), Vol. 3. Elsevier. https://doi.org/10.1016/B978-0-7020-5319-1.00016-5

# REPRO3 answers

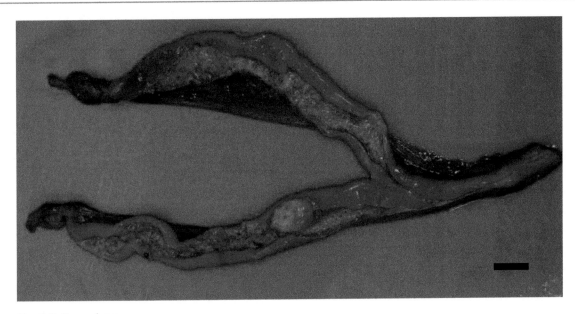

Fig. 9.5 **Bar = 1 cm.**

## 1. Describe any abnormalities

There are myriad tiny (mostly 1 mm diameter but up to ~1 cm diameter), thin-walled, fluid-filled, transparent cysts throughout the endometrium of both uterine horns.

## 2. Provide a diagnosis

Moderate diffuse cystic endometrial hyperplasia (CEH).

## 3. Briefly outline how progesterone and oestrogen influence the development of this lesion

Progesterone is the main hormone responsible for the hyperplasia that occurs in the endometrium of the dog and cat but there is still a reliance on previous oestrogen 'priming'. The endometrium hosts receptors for oestrogen. The interaction between these receptors and oestrogen triggers the formation of progesterone receptors which provide the route by which progesterone influences the endometrium to adopt a secretory path and become hyperplastic.

The importance of this condition lies in its association with pyometra since the latter condition often ultimately leads to anorexia, vomiting, polyuria and polydipsia, mainly due to toxaemia and likely also bacteraemia. Pyometra is induced by bacterial infections such as *E. coli* but the exact sequence of events is still not quite fully understood. Recent proposals suggest that bacteria can drive a progesterone-primed endometrium towards **both** pyometra **and** CEH, as opposed to CEH predisposing to bacterial infection and pyometra.[1]

### Reference

1  Schlafer, D. H., & Foster, R. A. (2016). Female genital system. In M. G. Maxie (Ed.), *Jubb, Kennedy and Palmer's pathology of domestic animals* (6th ed), Vol. 3. Elsevier. https://doi.org/10.1016/B978-0-7020-5319-1.00015-3

# REPRO4 answers

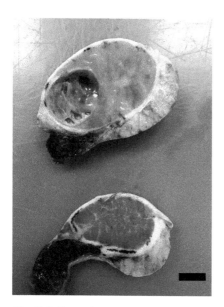

Fig. 9.6 Bar = 1 cm.

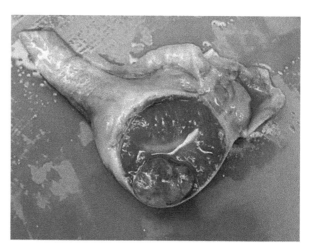

Fig. 9.6a Interstitial cell tumour, canine testis. The tan/orange colour is more easily appreciable in this case.

### 1.   Describe any abnormalities

Upper testis: The testicular parenchyma contains a well-demarcated, compressive and depressed mass that is pink/tan and cystic, measuring ~ 3 cm diameter.

   Lower testis: This testis is markedly reduced in size.

### 2.   Provide a diagnosis

Upper testis: Interstitial cell tumour (previously known as Leydig cell tumour).

Lower testis: Marked testicular atrophy.

### 3.   Which gross features justify your diagnosis?

Interstitial cell tumours are often well-demarcated but this is not a distinguishing feature. Best distinguishing features are (i) tan colour (often orange/tan – see Fig. 9.6a for better example); (ii) cystic areas (iii) areas of haemorrhage – not apparent here (Fig. 9.6b contains large areas of haemorrhage). The tan colour is probably due to the fact that Leydig cells are high in cholesterol required to make hormone (they are the testosterone-producing cells; for a similar reason, the adrenal cortex and its tumours are often a tan colour).

### Bonus question

Name the tumour on the left of Fig. 9.6b.

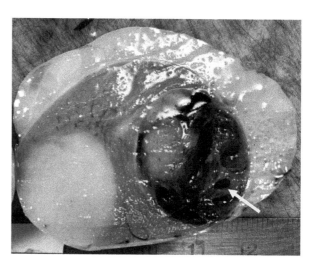

Fig. 9.6b This canine testis contains two tumours, which is not uncommon. The tumour on the right is an interstitial cell tumour, with the tan colour largely obscured by haemorrhage (the dark brown area) – small cystic structures are also just appreciable in the brown area (yellow arrow). Image credit: Dr Alex Malbon.

### Bonus answer

This is a testicular seminoma (smooth, homogenous and white; not fibrous enough for a Sertoli cell tumour).

# REPRO5 answers

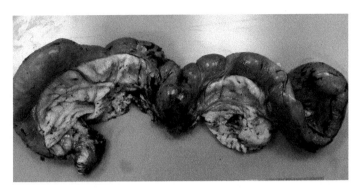

Fig. 9.7

## 1.  Describe any abnormalities

This is the uterus. It has been fixed which accounts for the diffuse, grey/purple colour of the serosal surface (prior to fixation it was deep red). Both uterine horns are markedly dilated and sacculated. Engorged vessels can also be seen through the serosal surface (see Fig. 9.7a). The dilation is due to accumulation of pus within the lumen of the uterine body and horns. The deposits of dark brown material over the surface are clotted blood secondary to the surgery.

## 2.  Provide a diagnosis

Severe diffuse pyometra (Confirms the clinical diagnosis!).

## 3.  Outline the pathogenesis of this condition and most likely reasons for this dog's (a) polyuria and (b) death

Pyometra literally means 'pus within the uterus'. In the bitch, this condition typically arises a few weeks after oestrus. The pathogenesis is still the subject of some debate but pyometra often occurs in conjunction with cystic endometrial hyperplasia (CEH) and is most commonly seen in middle-aged to older bitches. Progesterone priming of the endometrium can induce CEH and it was presumed that the associated secretions facilitated colonisation by bacteria and subsequent pyometra. Other studies have shown that, in the dioestrus/luteal phase, stimulation of the progesterone-primed endometrium (e.g. by mechanical trauma or bacteria) leads to CEH and pyometra. As a result, bacteria are a potential cause of concomitant CEH **and** pyometra (as opposed to pyometra resulting from bacterial infection of a uterus that already has CEH).[1]

a.  The pathogenesis of polyuria is not very well understood but it is postulated to be due to an immune based mechanism leading to a reduced capacity to concentrate urine. Affected animals may also develop membranoproliferative glomerulonephritis, which may also contribute.

b.  Death was most likely due to endotoxic shock. Pyometra may result in toxins/pus being released into the abdomen via the oviducts and/or perforation or rupture of the friable uterine wall. Both of these may result in peritonitis, sepsis/endotoxaemia and death (as in this case).

## Reference

1  Schlafer, D. H., & Foster, R. A. (2016). Female genital system. In M. G. Maxie (Ed.), *Jubb, Kennedy and Palmer's pathology of domestic animals* (6th ed), Vol. 3. Elsevier. https://doi.org/10.1016/B978-0-7020-5319-1.00015-3

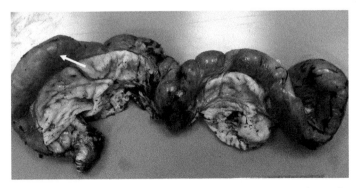

Fig. 9.7a **Fixed canine uterus. Arrow points to engorged vessels.**

# REPRO6 answers

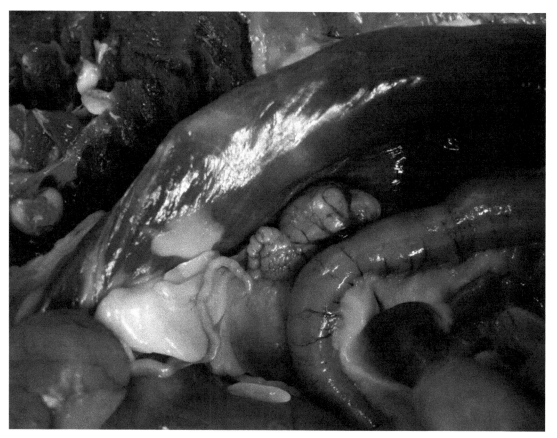

Fig. 9.8

## 1. Describe any abnormalities

Within the abdominal cavity, adjacent to a loop of small intestine, there is a small testis. This is slightly irregular and reduced in size.

## 2. Provide a diagnosis

Cryptorchidism with testicular hypoplasia.

## 3. This is now classified as a disorder of sexual development (DSD). Briefly outline:

### a) The cause of this condition

This is obviously congenital but it can be inherited in some breeds of dog (autosomal recessive) though is still largely idiopathic. It is more likely that the testis will be retained in the inguinal canal.

### b) Potential consequences

Testicular hypoplasia is usually present due to underdevelopment of the affected testis. The retained testis is also prone to neoplasia, particularly Sertoli (sustentacular) cell tumours and seminomas. Testicular torsion is another consequence. Testes should have descended fully by three months of age in the dog.[1]

## Reference

1   Foster, R. A. (2016). Male genital system. In In M. G. Maxie (Ed.), *Jubb, Kennedy and Palmer's pathology of domestic animals* (6th ed), Vol. 3. Elsevier. https://doi.org/10.1016/B978-0-7020-5319-1.00016-5

# REPRO7 answers

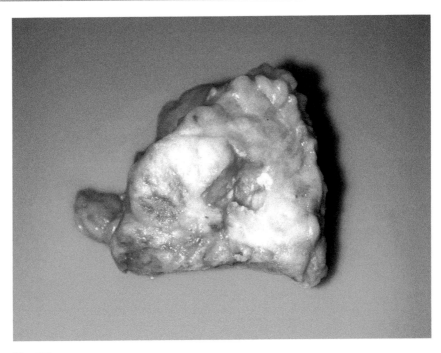

Fig. 9.9

## 1. Describe any abnormalities

This is the prostate gland but it is markedly distorted and misshapen, with its normal pale pink homogenous parenchyma replaced by a multinodular white mass, most obvious at the 12 o'clock to 3 o'clock position. The centre is cavitated and contains a small amount of yellow material (necrosis/pus).

## 2. Provide a diagnosis

Prostatic carcinoma.

> Necrotising prostatitis is a potential differential for tissue cavitation, necrosis and pus but it would not usually be associated with the formation of a multinodular white mass.

## 3. How would you expect this lesion to behave and how would you distinguish it from benign prostatic hyperplasia?

Prostatic carcinoma is potentially a very aggressive neoplasm with the capacity to metastasise via the lymphatic system to lymph nodes and distant organs, including bones. It may also spread transcoelomically within the peritoneal cavity, resulting in seeding of neoplastic epithelial cells on peritoneal surfaces, with an associated scirrhous reaction (also known as desmoplasia) that can lead to lymphatic obstruction and ascites. Other carcinomas that may be associated with this type of response are

carcinomas of urothelial, intestinal and pancreatic origin, among others.

Benign prostatic hyperplasia usually results in more even or uniform enlargement of the prostate gland (see Fig. 9.9a for comparison). The gland would appear diffusely enlarged with no cavitation, nodules or pus (unless otherwise inflamed). It is very common in male intact dogs and its development is influenced by testosterone.

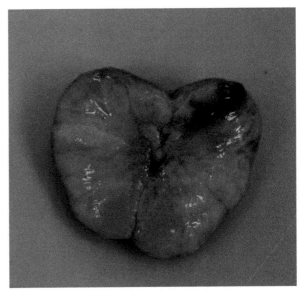

Fig. 9.9a Canine prostate with benign prostatic hyperplasia. There was also focal inflammation and haemorrhage.

# REPRO8 answers

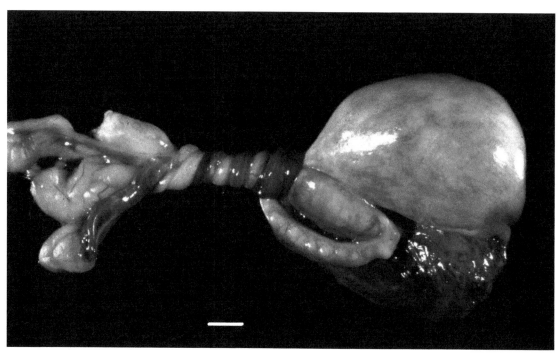

Fig. 9.10

## 1.  Describe any abnormalities
This is testis and spermatic cord in which the spermatic cord is tightly twisted around its central axis multiple times and the head of the epididymis is swollen, engorged and dark brown/red.

## 2.  Provide a diagnosis
Testicular torsion.

## 3.  Outline three other potential causes of scrotal swelling in the dog
Other potential causes include inflammation of scrotal contents, e.g. orchitis or epidymitis; scrotal hernia; neoplasia e.g. cutaneous or subcutaneous neoplasms such as mast cell tumour or scrotal vascular hamartoma; or testicular neoplasia (seminoma, sustentacular cell tumour*, interstitial cell tumour*, teratoma); abscess; haematoma; and seroma.

## Comment
Testicular torsion of the descended testis is rare in the dog and most cases arise in retained testes, presumably because they lie free within the abdomen and there is an increased risk of neoplasia, which adds bulk or volume to facilitate the torsion.[1] When torsion occurs in descended testes, it is not usually associated with underlying testicular neoplasia. The torsion of the spermatic cord vasculature leads to engorgement of the epididymis and eventually venous infarction.[2]

*Sustentacular cell tumours were previously known as Sertoli cell tumours and interstitial cell tumours were previously also known as Leydig cell tumours.

## References
1  Foster, R. A. (2016). Male genital system. In M. G. Maxie (Ed.), *Jubb, Kennedy and Palmer's pathology of domestic animals* (6th ed), Vol. 3. Elsevier. https://doi.org/10.1016/B978-0-7020-5319-1.00016-5

2  Boza, S., de Membiela, F., Navarro, A., Escobar, M. T., Soler, M., & Agut, A. (2011). What is your diagnosis? Testicular torsion. *Journal of the American Veterinary Medical Association, 238*(1), 37–38. https://doi.org/10.2460/javma.238.1.37

# Central nervous system cases

**10**

# CNS1

## Topics

Lesion recognition

Practical technique

Generation of pathological differential diagnoses lists

## History

A 2Y old, female neutered Mastiff dog arrived at a specialist veterinary hospital in cardiorespiratory arrest. Attempts at resuscitation were unsuccessful and the body was necropsied. The clinical history had been vague, comprising inappetence, lethargy and 'looking for places to hide'. Urine analysis, haematology and serum biochemistry were all within normal limits. Figs 10.1–10.3 illustrate the most significant necropsy finding. The dotted line in Fig. 10.2 highlights the level at which the section in Fig. 10.3 (fixed tissue) was taken.

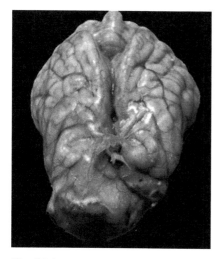

Fig. 10.1

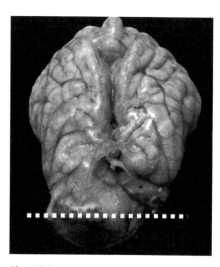

Fig. 10.2

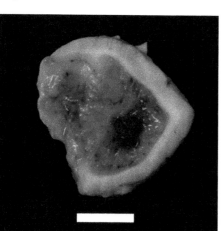

Fig. 10.3 Bar = 1 cm.

## Questions

1. Describe any abnormalities.
2. Provide a diagnosis.
3. Outline how you would sample and prepare this brain to facilitate a histological diagnosis.

# CNS2

## Topics

Lesion recognition

Generation of pathological differential diagnoses lists

## History

This 3Y old, male intact Red Setter had been rescued 10 days previously, so its history was mostly unknown, although it was fully vaccinated. Ataxia was noted at the time of rescue, with progression over 24–48 hours. At time of clinical presentation to a veterinary neurologist the dog was very depressed with a wide-base stance in all four limbs, and truncal swaying. There was an absent menace response in the left eye, but palpebral and pupillary light reflexes were normal. The clinical diagnosis was multifocal CNS disease involving the cerebellum. The dog was euthanised and submitted for necropsy. The brain was grossly normal when first removed from the skull but not when sectioned post fixation.

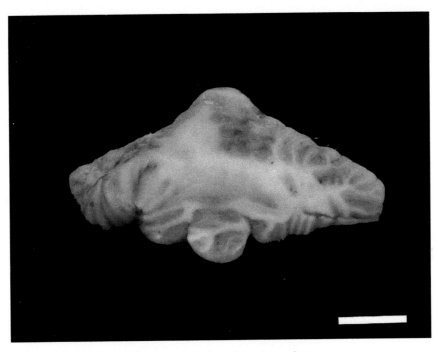

Fig. 10.4  Canine cerebellum, coronal section. Bar = 1 cm.

## Questions

1. Describe any abnormalities.
2. Provide a diagnosis.
3. Provide some differential diagnoses for multifocal CNS disease in the dog. What other information would help?

# CNS3

## Topic covered

**Lesion recognition**

## History

An 11Y old, male neutered, domestic shorthair cat presented with sudden onset seizures of increasing frequency over a two-week period. The seizures became refractory to treatment and the owners elected euthanasia. Necropsy confirmed the suspected space-occupying lesion (Fig. 10.5).

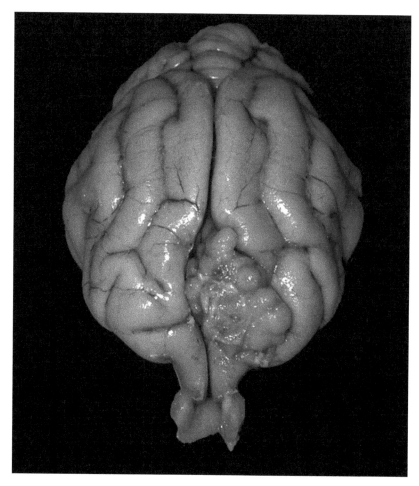

Fig. 10.5

## Questions

1. Describe any abnormalities.
2. Provide a diagnosis.
3. What is the most common primary brain tumour in the cat?

# CNS4

## Topics

Lesion recognition

Integration of pathological findings with clinical aspects

Prioritisation of findings

## History

A 9Y old, male German Shepherd Dog was euthanised due to sudden onset unilateral hind limb paresis that occurred after a road accident. The dog was otherwise bright and responsive but had urinary incontinence.

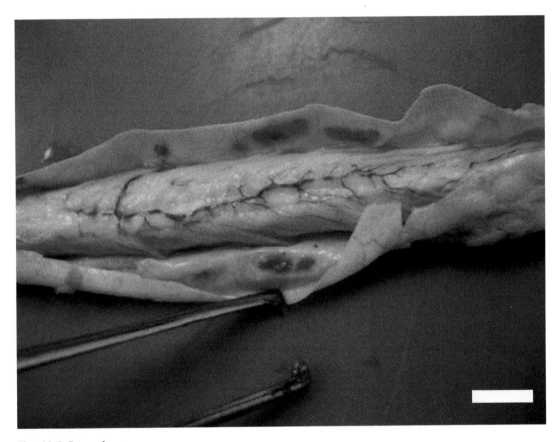

Fig. 10.6  Bar = 1 cm.

## Questions

1. Describe any abnormalities.
2. Provide a diagnosis.
3. Outline the clinical significance of the lesion(s) in terms of this dog's presentation.

# CNS5

## Topics

**Lesion recognition**

**Prioritisation of findings**

**Approach to difficult cases**

## History

A 6Y old, male neutered Standard Poodle presented with sudden onset seizure activity that progressed to status epilepticus and was refractory to treatment. Biochemistry and haematology were within normal limits and the dog had no known access to toxins. Due to the lack of response to treatment, the dog was euthanised. Fig. 10.7 shows the brain from this dog pre fixation.

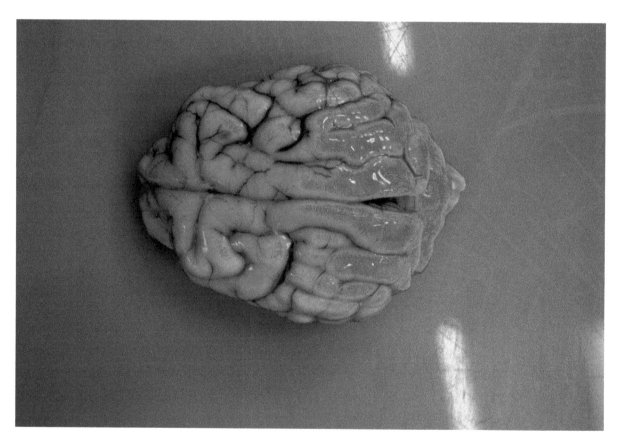

Fig. 10.7

## Questions

1. Describe any abnormalities.
2. Provide a diagnosis.
3. What considerations and actions would you pursue during this necropsy to try to reach a satisfactory diagnosis?

# CNS6

## Topics

Lesion recognition

Generation of pathological differential diagnoses lists

Pathogenesis

## History

A 9Y old, female neutered Labradoodle presented for necropsy following elective euthanasia. A mass had been identified on computed tomography (CT) following referral to a neurologist. As expected, the most significant necropsy finding was in the brain (Fig. 10.8).

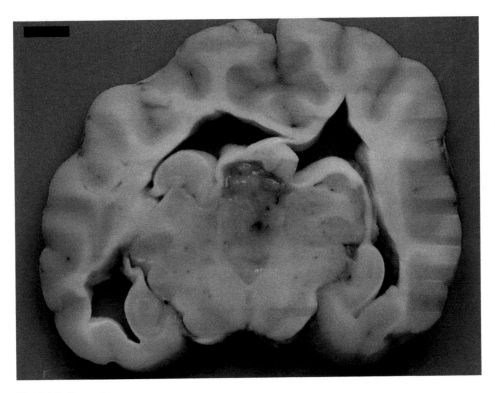

Fig. 10.8  Bar = 1 cm.

## Questions

1. Describe any abnormalities.
2. Provide a diagnosis.
3. Outline the pathogenesis of the hydrocephalus in this case.

# CNS7

## Topics

**Lesion recognition**

**Integration of pathological findings with clinical aspects**

## History

The image in Fig. 10.9 depicts the most significant gross necropsy finding in a 4Y old, male neutered Bichon Frise.

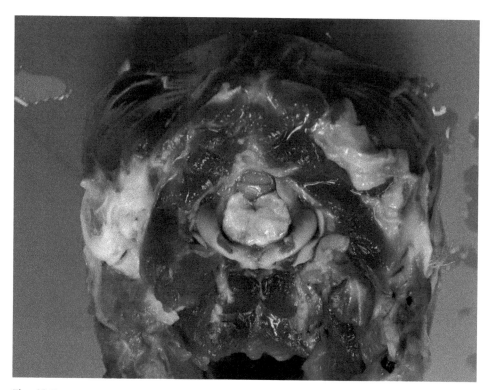

Fig. 10.9

## Questions

1. Describe any abnormalities.
2. Provide a diagnosis.
3. What is the potential significance of this lesion?

# CNS8

## Topics

Practical technique

Common artefacts and pitfalls

## History

This brain originated from a 2Y old, male domestic shorthair cat that was the focus of a cruelty case being pursued by local authorities. For legal reasons, the body had been stored in a freezer for 6 weeks prior to submission for necropsy.

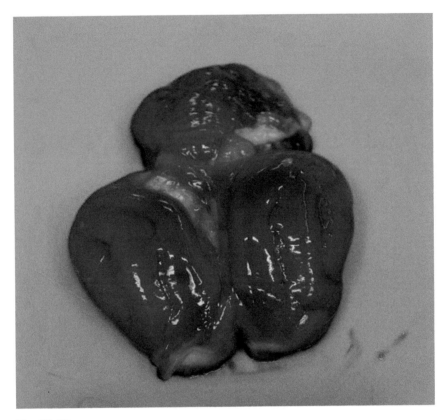

Fig. 10.10

## Questions

1. Describe any abnormalities.
2. Provide a diagnosis.
3. How diagnostically useful or relevant is this brain?

# CNS9

## Topics

Lesion recognition

Prioritisation of findings

Pathogenesis

## History

This is the brain from a 7Y old, male neutered Bulldog that had been euthanised due to progressive neurological disease.

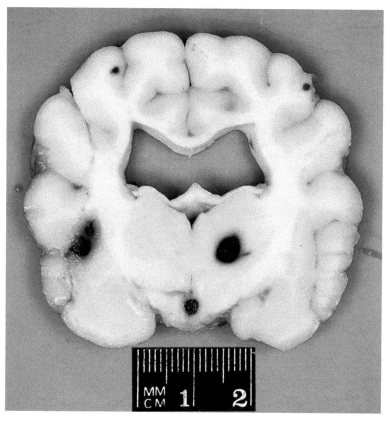

Fig. 10.11 Image credit: Alistair Cox.

## Questions

1. Describe any abnormalities.
2. Provide a diagnosis.
3. (a) Why is this most likely to be metastatic rather than primary neoplasia?
   (b) What is the likely pathogenesis of the hydrocephalus?

# CNS10

## Topics

Lesion recognition

Common artefacts and pitfalls

Prioritisation of findings

## History

The brain in Fig. 10.12 was removed from a 10Y old, male neutered Bulldog that had a clinical history of brachycephalic obstructive airway syndrome and had died at home.

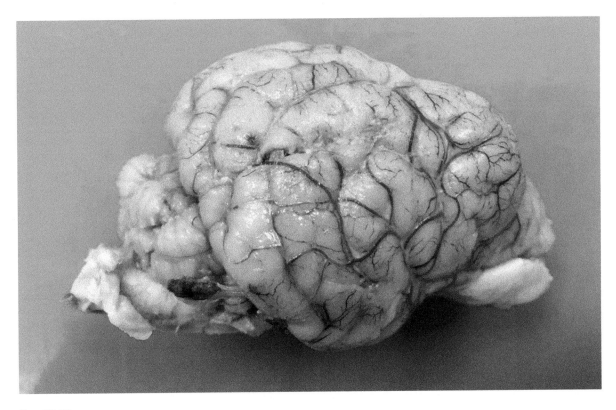

Fig. 10.12

## Questions

1. Describe any abnormalities.
2. Provide a diagnosis.
3. Briefly outline necropsy findings that would support vulnerability to brachycephalic obstructive airway syndrome (BOAS) in the dog. How do the changes in Fig. 10.12 contribute to BOAS?

# CNS1 answers

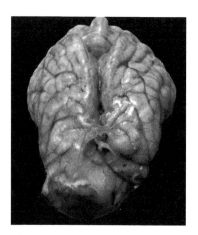

Fig. 10.1

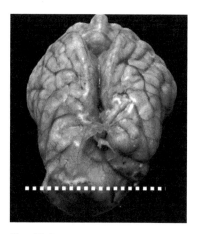

Fig. 10.2

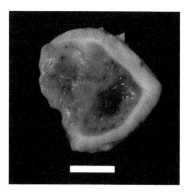

Fig. 10.3  Bar = 1 cm.

## 1.   Describe any abnormalities

The rostral aspect of the right frontal cortex contains a well-demarcated but irregular, ~2.5 cm diameter, soft, fluctuant, gelatinous, grey mass that is intramedullary (i.e. within the parenchyma). The mass is also locally invasive, encroaching on the rostral-most aspect of the left cerebrum. In Fig. 10.3 the mass has a white rim and grey/black areas within (post-fixation areas of haemorrhage). It is very slightly compressive.

## 2.   Provide a diagnosis

This is a cerebral glioma. Histopathology confirmed an oligodendroglioma. A solitary mass within the parenchyma of the canine brain is much more likely to be a primary than a secondary (metastatic) brain tumour. This location, together with the grey colour and slightly gelatinous texture, is supportive of a glioma. The most commonly reported primary brain tumour in both dogs and cats is the meningioma, but it is generally a surface tumour. Gliomas are the next most frequent primary tumour, followed by the much less frequently reported ependymoma and choroid plexus tumour (the latter two tend to arise in the ventricles). Primitive neuroectodermal

tumours are rare and a metastatic neoplasm would be more likely to be multifocal. The young age of this dog is more atypical since gliomas tend to arise in older dogs, but this does not exclude neoplasia. The other main differential is a granuloma. It would be very unusual for a granuloma to present as a solitary, grossly appreciable mass in the dog but it would also be a straightforward histological rule-out.

## 3.   Outline how you would sample and prepare this brain to facilitate a histological diagnosis

Fix the brain in a large container of 10% neutral buffered formalin (NBF) for at least seven days prior to sectioning. Brain (and spinal cord) should not be sectioned until adequately fixed as the tissue is too soft and sectioning will lead to tissue damage and artefact. Some prefer to fix in higher concentrations of NBF but 10% works well in our experience. If there is the suspicion of an infectious process, you might consider taking a very small sample of the lesion for bacterial/fungal culture – do that before fixing.

> See more details in Chapter 1, 'Brain trimming guide'.

> TIP
>
> In the event that you decide to send an entire brain to a veterinary pathology laboratory, and since it is prohibited to send large volumes of formalin in the post, we recommend that you fix the brain first in a large volume of formalin, then send it as one organ to the laboratory (i.e. do not section it). You can still wrap it in paper towels soaked in formalin, double bag and place in a robust container surrounded by absorbent material, such as cotton wool.

# CNS2 answers

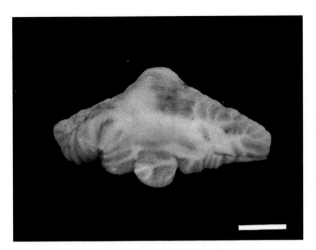

Fig. 10.4 Canine cerebellum, coronal section.
Bar = 1 cm.

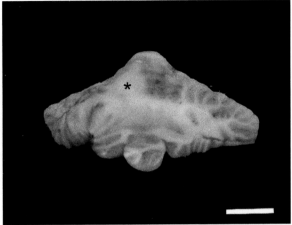

Fig. 10.4a Canine cerebellum with a localised area of glial scarring (*) obscuring the grey/white interface.

## 1.   Describe any abnormalities

There is focal replacement of the cerebellar parenchyma on the left side by an ill-defined, approximately 5 mm diameter, smooth, white lesion, with associated loss of distinction at the grey-white interface (see Fig. 10.4a).

## 2.   Provide a diagnosis

Severe, focally extensive, necrotising, cerebellar encephalitis.

## 3.   Provide some differential diagnoses for multifocal CNS disease in the dog. What other information would help?

Individual aetiologies are myriad! They are also well detailed in relevant veterinary neurology and pathology textbooks.[1,2] However, infectious diseases include canine distemper, rabies, pseudorabies, West Nile virus, tick-borne encephalitis, protozoal, bacterial and fungal encephalomyelitis. Canine herpesvirus type 1 only occurs in neonates. Bear in mind that some toy breeds as predisposed to breed-related encephalitis (e.g. Maltese and Yorkshire terriers). A vaccination history is always very helpful and, since some of these diseases do not occur in the UK (rabies, West Nile virus), travel history would also be useful. In a rescue case like this, such information may not be freely available. However, we did know this dog was vaccinated. Granulomatous meningoencephalitis generally presents as multifocal CNS disease clinically but is still considered idiopathic. Metastatic neoplasia could also present as multifocal CNS disease (e.g. lymphoma, metastatic haemangiosarcoma).

Histopathology of this case confirmed chronic active meningoencephalitis with regionally extensive cerebellar encephalomalacia, glial scarring and intralesional protozoal cysts. Serology titres indicated exposure to *Neospora caninum* so, collectively, histopathology and serology were most compatible with CNS neospora infection. For many of the above infectious diseases (particularly those of a viral aetiology), the brain would be grossly normal and histopathology would be required to reach a diagnosis. Most viral and protozoal diseases in the CNS cause non-suppurative (i.e. lymphoplasmacytic) inflammation that is only appreciable microscopically. Grossly appreciable lesions such as those in this case tend to suggest more severe inflammation and/or malacia, or perhaps glial scarring. The white area denoted by the asterisk in Fig 10.5 was dominated microscopically by glial scar tissue, the CNS equivalent of fibrosis.

## References

1   Cantile, C., & Youssef, S. (2016). Nervous system. In M. G. Maxie (Ed.), *Jubb, Kennedy and Palmer's pathology of domestic animals* (6th ed), Vol. 1. Elsevier. https://doi.org/10.1016/B978-0-7020-5317-7.00004-7

2   Summers, B. A,, Cummings, J. F., & DeLahunta, A. (1995). *Veterinary neuropathology*. Mosby.

# CNS3 answers

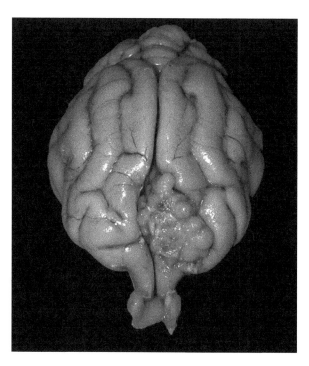

Fig. 10.5

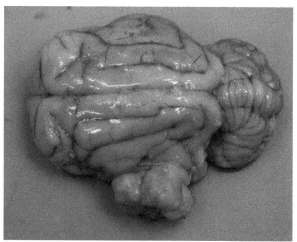

Fig. 10.5a **Feline meningioma protruding from the lateral aspect of the left cerebral hemisphere.**

## 1. Describe any abnormalities

A pedunculated, 2 cm × 1 cm diameter, grey, multilobulated and mildly compressive mass with a smooth surface protrudes from the falx cerebri in the central longitudinal fissure, veering towards the left side of the brain.

## 2. Provide a diagnosis

Cerebral meningioma.

## 3. What is the most common primary brain tumour in the cat?

This one – meningioma. This is also the most common tumour overall arising in the feline brain (including secondary tumours).[1,2] Studies indicate that meningioma accounts for well over 50% of primary brain tumours in the cat.[2] From the few studies there are assessing large numbers of cases, lymphoma is consistently the second most common form of neoplasia.[1,2] Meningomas are usually solitary, though there may be more than one concurrently.[1] They tend to be compressive and non-invasive (unlike their canine equivalent which is more likely to be invasive).[1] Like most primary brain tumours, they are non-metastatic. The falx cerebri is a common site for these but they can occur anywhere on the surface of the brain, e.g. Fig. 10.5a.

## References

1 Zaki, F. A., & Hurvitz, A. I. (1976). Spontaneous neoplasms of the central nervous system of the cat. *Journal of Small Animal Practice*, 17(12), 773–782. https://doi.org/10.1111/j.1748-5827.1976.tb06943.x

2 Troxel, M. T., Vite, C. H., Van Winkle, T. J., Newton, A. L., Tiches, D., Dayrell-Hart, B., Kapatkin, A. S., Shofer, F. S., & Steinberg, S. A. (2003). Feline intracranial neoplasia: Retrospective review of 160 cases (1985–2001) (1985–2001). *Journal of Veterinary Internal Medicine*, 17(6), 850–859. https://doi.org/10.1111/j.1939-1676.2003.tb02525.x

# CNS4 answers

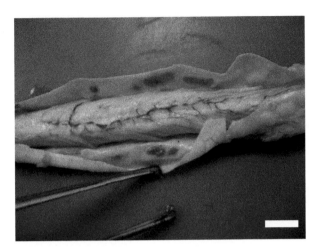

Fig. 10.6 **Bar = 1 cm.**

## 1.  Describe any abnormalities

There are multiple (<10) brown, slightly raised, oval, well-demarcated plaques within the dura mater. They range in length up to approximately 1 cm and measure approximately 3–4 mm wide.

## 2.  Provide a diagnosis

Dural ossification.

## 3.  Outline the clinical significance of the lesion(s) in terms of this dog's presentation

Dural ossification (also known as ossifying pachymeningitis) is a common incidental finding more commonly seen in older dogs. It has no clinical significance in this case so it would be important to progress as normal, with examination of the musculoskeletal system, brain and spinal cord macroscopically with follow-up fixation to allow histopathological assessment and a search for a more significant lesion.

In this case, there were no additional macroscopic findings at time of necropsy. The non-progressive presentation following trauma may be quite suggestive of disc protrusion or a vascular aetiology e.g. fibrocartilaginous embolic myelopathy (depending on degree of injury these may present as paresis or paralysis). Disc protrusion would be identifiable following removal of the spinal cord, but a more thorough search for a spinal infarct, vascular disease or embolic cartilage in spinal vessels would be an important part of the diagnostic process. This would require retention of the full length of the spinal cord, followed by thorough histological assessment of multiple sections of spinal cord from different levels. Wallerian-like degeneration will mainly occur in the dorsolateral funiculi of the spinal cord cranial to the point of injury whereas, caudal to the point of injury, such changes are mainly in the ventrolateral region. It would also be important to be open-minded as to the possibility of other lesions such as a vertebral fracture, limbs or pelvic fracture, or underlying concomitant soft tissue injury involving muscles, nerves or joints (paresis may be due to nervous or muscular system dysfunction).

# CNS5 answers

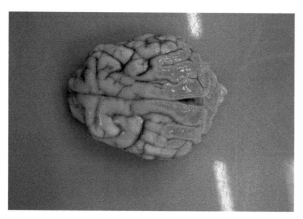

Fig. 10.7

## 1.　Describe any abnormalities

This is essentially a grossly normal brain. Note that it is common for the brain to be grossly normal in dogs and cats presenting with central nervous system disease – histopathology is always indicated.

## 2.　Provide a diagnosis

Grossly normal.

## 3.　What considerations and actions would you pursue during this necropsy to try to reach a satisfactory diagnosis?

As the history is not supportive of an extracranial (i.e. metabolic or toxic cause) for the seizures, they are likely to be the result of intracranial disease, so the brain is the focus of the necropsy. Seizures are caused by spontaneous depolarisation of intracranial neurons. There are many causes but broad underlying intracranial causes are (i) structural (ii) idiopathic epilepsy (i.e. genetic) and (iii) epilepsy of unknown cause.[1,2] When a lesion is not grossly apparent in the freshly removed brain, it is always worth collecting a fresh sample for culture and even retaining a small piece frozen. An unobtrusive area to sample for fresh tissue is the pyriform lobe on one side. Then the brain should be handled and packaged as outlined in case CNS1 unless you are responsible for the further processing of the tissues (see below).

Pathological evaluation will include coronal (transverse) sectioning of the brain at approximately 5 mm intervals to try to identify any space-occupying lesion (tumour, haematoma, abscess, granuloma); to assess the ventricular system (and rule out hydrocephalus); and to check for other lesions such as haemorrhage, malacia, congenital lesions and cerebellar herniation – the latter usually indicates increased intracranial pressure and/or oedema. Representative sections must be examined histologically (see Chapter 1, 'Brain trimming guide'). This process is usually able to exclude or identify a structural reason for seizures if conducted thoroughly. Histopathology is particularly important to identify (or rule out) any underlying infectious or degenerative disease process, vascular disease, infarction or infiltrative neoplasia.

At time of necropsy for any animal with seizures, it is also important to check the head/skull for evidence of trauma (or indeed any other abnormalities) and to exclude a neoplastic process that may have metastasised to the brain. Good examples of malignancies that have a propensity to spread to the CNS include haemangiosarcoma, melanoma and mammary carcinoma. Underlying metabolic disease can be supported by antemortem haematology and biochemistry which may at least provide some pointers (as mentioned in the history, they were normal in this case). Potential metabolic causes include liver disease, renal failure, pancreatic disease, paraneoplastic syndrome or endocrine disease involving thyroid, parathyroid, pituitary, and/or adrenal glands (so the broader necropsy is still very important). Finally, fresh samples of various internal organs should be retained, appropriate for toxicological evaluation, since certain drugs and heavy metals (lead) can trigger seizures. We generally collect a panel to include liver, kidney, blood (clotted or unclotted), urine and stomach contents as a minimum. Lung and fat can be useful.

This would be a reasonable approach in any dog (or cat) that presents with neurological signs and in which the brain is grossly normal, bearing in mind that, depending on clinical signs, spinal cord may need to be evaluated too.

## References

1　Ekenstedt, K. J., & Oberbauer, A. M. (2013). Inherited epilepsy in dogs. *Topics in Companion Animal Medicine, 28*(2), 51–58. https://doi.org/10.1053/j.tcam.2013.07.001, PubMed: 24070682

2　Muñana, K. R. (2017). Seizures. In S. J. Ettinger, E. C. Feldman, & E. Cote (Eds.) *Textbook of veterinary internal medicine: Diseases of the dog and the cat* (pp. 142–144). Saunders.

# CNS6 answers

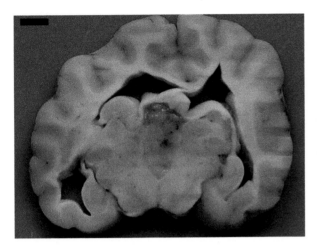

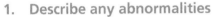

Fig. 10.8 Bar = 1 cm.

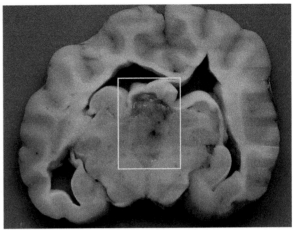

Fig. 10.8a Canine brain with grey mass filling the third ventricle.

## 1.   Describe any abnormalities

The brain parenchyma is generally distorted, leading to asymmetry and elevation of the fornix of the hippocampus. The third ventricle is dilated and filled with a soft, slightly gelatinous, grey mass that measures up to approximately 2.5 cm × 1.5 cm (see yellow rectangle in Fig. 10.8a). The lateral ventricles are moderately dilated bilaterally. In the plane of section perpendicular to this image, the tumour extended caudally from the rostral thalamus into the mesencephalic aqueduct and on to the pons.

## 2.   Provide a diagnosis

It is difficult to be definitive in this case without knowledge of histopathological findings but you should at least have some differentials with a hierarchy of likelihood based on location. The tumour is within the third ventricle, so the two main differentials are an ependymoma or a choroid plexus tumour. Ependymal cells line the ventricular system while the choroid plexus comprises modified ependymal cells which filter blood to create cerebrospinal fluid. Histopathology is required to make the diagnosis, sometimes supported by immunohistochemistry. This was confirmed as an ependymoma histologically.

**Diagnosis:** Ependymoma with moderate bilateral hydrocephalus

## 3.   Outline the pathogenesis of the hydrocephalus in this case

Hydrocephalus implies an increased amount of cerebrospinal fluid (CSF) *in the cranial cavity*. When within the ventricles this is termed *internal hydrocephalus*. The space-occupying effects of this mass would have caused obstruction of the third ventricle and mesencephalic aqueduct, leading to build-up of fluid rostral to the blockage (the lateral ventricles) and subsequent dilation of the lateral ventricles. Over time, pressure would lead to loss of brain parenchyma too.

### Pathway of CSF production:

CSF is produced by the choroid plexus cells within the ventricles and passes through the lateral ventricles → third ventricle → fourth ventricle → CSF flows out through apertures on the lateral aspect of brain stem → flows over surface of brain in the subarachnoid space → resorbed into the blood by the arachnoid villi.

# CNS7 answers

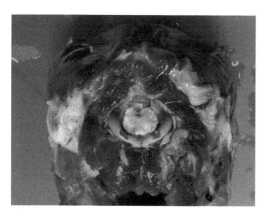

Fig. 10.9

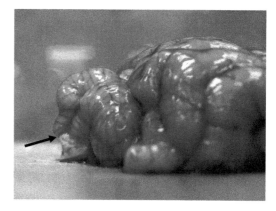

Fig. 10.9b **The lateral view shows 'lipping' of the vermis over the compressed medulla (arrow).**

## 1. Describe any abnormalities

In Fig. 10.9 the ventral vermis of the cerebellum is (abnormally) visible at the foramen magnum and there is associated downward displacement and compression of the medulla. See also Figs 10.9a and 10.9b below.

## 2. Provide a diagnosis

Cerebellar herniation at foramen magnum.

## 3. What is the potential significance of this lesion?

Herniation of the brain is an indicator of increased intracranial pressure. The skull is obviously rigid with no room for manoeuvre if it is swollen or compressed. The only way it can avoid further damage is to prolapse at several points within the cranial vault. Herniation may occur in five recognised locations in the skull, but the foramen magnum is the location we most commonly see and it is one of the two most clinically significant locations (the other is at the tentorium cerebelli, so-called subtentorial herniation).[1-3]

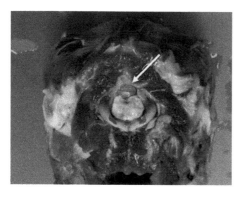

Fig. 10.9a **Cerebellar herniation – arrow points to the protruding cerebellar vermis – we should not be able to see it at this stage of the necropsy.**

Causes of increased intracranial pressure may include inflammation, a space-occupying lesion (including neoplasia), inflammation, haemorrhage / haematoma or oedema. The significance of this lesion is that consequent compression of the medulla can result in suppression of respiration and death.

## Comment

Note that herniation of the cerebellum is a feature of Chiari-like syndrome in the Cavalier King Charles Spaniel, due to a malformation (hypoplasia) of the caudal cranial fossa.[4] Techniques such as magnetic resonance imaging mean that this diagnosis is typically now made premortem, but care should still be taken at necropsy since the herniated cerebellum may be overlooked if the cap of the skull is removed without specific attention to the affected area.

## References

1 Minato, S., Cherubini, G. B., Della Santa, D., Salvadori, S., & Baroni, M. (2021). Incidence and type of brain herniation associated with intracranial meningioma in dogs and cats. *Journal of Veterinary Medical Science, 83*(2), 267–273. https://doi.org/10.1292/jvms.20-0111

2 Lewis, M. J., Olby, N. J., Early, P. J., Mariani, C. L., Muñana, K. R., Seiler, G. S., & Griffith, E. H. (2016). Clinical and diagnostic imaging features of brain herniation in dogs and cats. *Journal of Veterinary Internal Medicine, 30*(5), 1672–1680. https://doi.org/10.1111/jvim.14526

3 Summers, B. A,, Cummings, J. F., & DeLahunta, A. (1995). *Veterinary neuropathology*. Mosby.

4 Carrera, I., Dennis, R., Mellor, D. J., Penderis, J., & Sullivan, M. (2009). Use of magnetic resonance imaging for morphometric analysis of the caudal cranial fossa in Cavalier King Charles Spaniels. *American Journal of Veterinary Research, 70*(3), 340–345. https://doi.org/10.2460/ajvr.70.3.340

# CNS8 answers

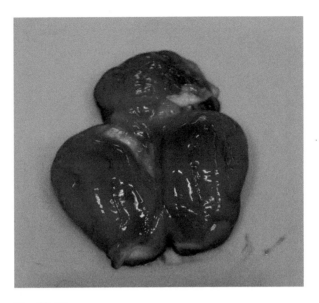

Fig. 10.10

## 1. Describe any abnormalities

The brain is extremely flaccid and diffusely discoloured red/pink. There is loss of distinction of the sulci in particular.

> Note that this brain is not fixed – a fresh, unfrozen brain is normally white to pale pink and slightly soft but the cerebral hemispheres do not flatten and separate like this.

## 2. Provide a diagnosis

This is an artefact, resulting from the freeze/thaw process. It is not a lesion.

## 3. How diagnostically useful or relevant is this brain?

This brain could still provide some information and should still be fixed, especially in a cruelty case, where someone further along the legal process may want to know if it was examined and, if so, how thoroughly. It will still be reliable for exclusion or identification of a grossly appreciable space-occupying lesion. A portion can also be retained for toxicology if necessary (and even re-frozen). However, it is less useful for bacterial or fungal culture as the freezing process will impact on the viability of some organisms. Freezing is also highly detrimental to microscopic structure and renders the organ and tissues much less diagnostically useful for histopathology (not just the brain, all organs and tissues). Refer to GIT8 for more details.

> TIP
> **NEVER** freeze the body if you can possibly avoid it …
>     … and …
> **NEVER EVER** freeze the body in a neurological case !!
> In reality, there may be times when you have absolutely no choice, but this is the rule, whenever possible.
>     If there is really no option other than to freeze, make sure everyone concerned is made aware of the significant drawbacks. There is a high risk of not reaching a reliable diagnosis, particularly in neurological cases, perhaps with the exception of trauma-induced injuries.

# CNS9 answers

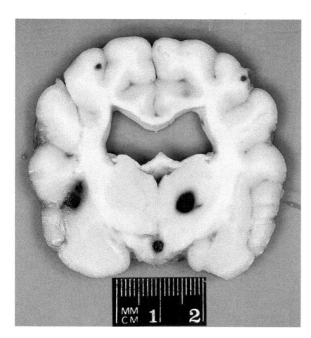

Fig. 10.11 Image credit: Alistair Cox.

## 1. Describe any abnormalities

There are multifocal (n=5) well-demarcated, dark red/black lesions scattered randomly in the parenchyma of both sides of the brain, ranging from oval to irregular and from 1 mm diameter to ~8 mm × 5 mm. Both lateral ventricles are also moderately dilated.

## 2. Provide a diagnosis

There are two lesions:

a. Metastatic haemangiosarcoma (metastatic melanoma is a reasonable differential although we might expect the lesions to be even more densely black).

b. Moderate bilateral hydrocephalus.

## 3.

### (a) Why is this most likely to be metastatic rather than primary neoplasia?

The multifocal and random pattern suggests secondary neoplasia that has reached the brain via the haematogenous

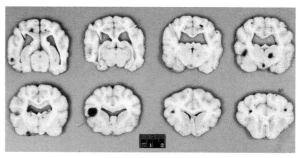

Fig. 10.11a Canine brain, serially sectioned, with metastatic hamangiosarcoma and moderate bilateral hydrocephalus. Image credit: Alistair Cox.

route (see Fig. 10.11a which shows how dispersed this tumour was). The tumour deposits also vary in size, suggesting that they arrived at different times. Primary brain neoplasia is generally solitary and, while primary cerebral haemangiosarcoma is theoretically possible (and has been reported[1]), it is extremely rare. Common sites of origin for haemangiosarcoma are the right atrium, the spleen and liver. Common sites of origin for malignant melanoma are the oral cavity and subungual area of the digit. Only about 15% of primary cutaneous melanomas are potentially malignant.

### (b) What is the likely pathogenesis of the hydrocephalus?

The hydrocephalus is most likely pre-existing. Brachycephalic breeds are more predisposed to hydrocephalus and it is often incidental in such cases. If a tumour deposit is lodged somewhere important to the CSF flow then hydrocephalus could feasibly occur secondary to the haemangiosarcoma (e.g. in or around the mesencephalic aqueduct).

### Reference

1 Gabor, L. J., & Vanderstichel, R. V. (2006). Primary cerebral hemangiosarcoma in a 6-week-old dog. *Veterinary Pathology*, *43*(5), 782–784. https://doi.org/10.1354/vp.43-5-782

# CNS10 answers

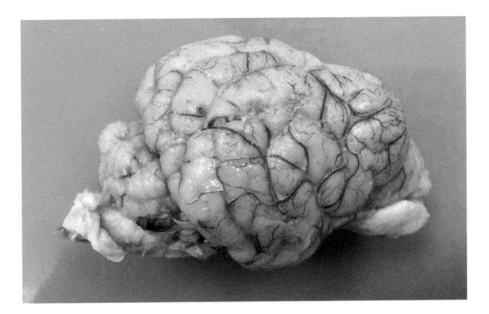

Fig 10.12

## 1.   Describe any abnormalities

The image shows the right side of the brain, mainly the cerebrum, with cerebellum and brainstem on the left. There is linear deposition of grey/white material in the cerebral sulci, generally following the path of the blood vessels. There is also a small, well-demarcated black focus on the ventral aspect of the right side of the cerebellum, measuring ~1 cm × 0.5 cm.

## 2.   Provide a diagnosis
   a.  Leptomeningeal fibrosis.
   b.  Mild focal leptomeningeal melanosis.

## 3.   Briefly outline necropsy findings that would support vulnerability to brachycephalic obstructive airway syndrome (BOAS) in the dog. How do the changes in Fig. 10.12 contribute to BOAS?

Necropsy findings that support BOAS are:

- tracheal hypoplasia; elongated and thickened soft palate; stenotic nares; enlarged tongue; enlarged and/or everted tonsils[1]
- everted laryngeal saccules and laryngeal collapse may also be significantly involved although this is more controversial.[1]

The changes in Fig. 10.12 do not contribute at all to BOAS. Leptomeningeal fibrosis has no clinical significance. It is age related and arises due to deposition of fibrous connective tissue in the leptomeninges. It may be mistaken for pus (hence this is a potential 'pitfall') but it cannot be removed – pus can be dislodged or smeared with your finger (an impression smear would usually confirm pus easily by demonstrating lots of neutrophils). Pus will also tend to gravitate ventrally rather than accumulating dorsally. So, this is not meningitis.

The small area of black discolouration within the cerebellar leptomeninges is simply a localised increase in melanin. It is not a true lesion but is similar to areas of melanin deposition on mucosal surfaces or the intimal surface of large blood vessels. It is not a pathological change or even an artefact, but normal for the affected individual.

## Reference

1   Krainer, D., & Dupré, G. (2022). Brachycephalic obstructive airway syndrome. *Veterinary Clinics of North America: Small Animal Practice*, *52*(3), 749–780. https://doi.org/10.1016/j.cvsm.2022.01.013

# Endocrine cases

11

# END1

## Topics

- Lesion recognition
- Pathogenesis
- Integration of pathological findings with clinical aspects

## History

A 9Y old, female neutered German Shepherd Dog presented for necropsy following a prolonged period of treatment for hyperadrenocorticism and, ultimately, euthanasia on welfare grounds, due to failure to respond to treatment. The most pertinent findings are illustrated in Fig. 11.1.

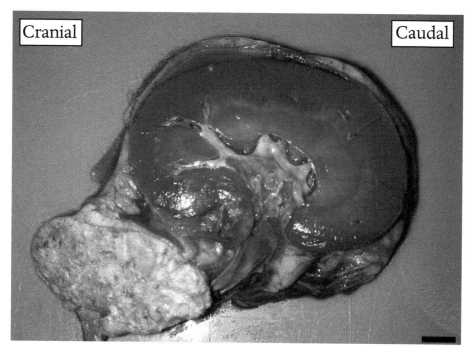

Fig. 11.1 Bar = 1 cm.

## Questions

1. Describe any abnormalities.
2. Provide a diagnosis.
3. Why might there be cortical atrophy of the contralateral adrenal gland?

# END2

## Topics

Lesion recognition

Integration of pathological findings with clinical aspects

Pathogenesis

Practical technique

## History

A 7Y old, male neutered domestic shorthair cat was presented for necropsy following euthanasia. Clinical signs had included vomiting, anorexia, depression, polyuria and polydipsia, with intermittent and generalised weakness. The main necropsy finding is illustrated in Fig. 11.2 but there were also multiple slightly gritty to chalky, white plaques scattered throughout the subcutaneous fat and fascia of the ventral abdomen, as well as within some limb muscles. These plaques were flat and measured up to 1 cm diameter.

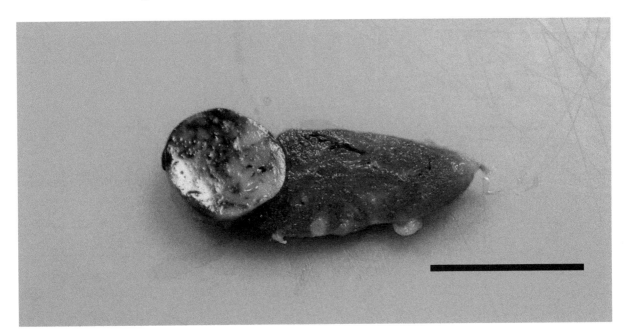

Fig. 11.2  Bar = 1 cm.

## Questions

1. Describe any abnormalities.
2. Provide a diagnosis.
3. This is an example of primary hyperparathyroidism. Outline (a) the normal function of the parathyroid gland and (b) the pathogenesis of primary hyperparathyroidism and how it impacts on pathological features of this case.

# END3

## Topics

Lesion recognition

Integration of pathological findings with clinical aspects

Pathogenesis

## History

A 6Y old, female neutered Boxer presented with a six-month history of progressive lethargy, inappetance, polyuria (PU) and polydipsia (PD). Urine analysis results were normal. Haematology, biochemistry and ancillary test results indicated hyperglycaemia, hypercholesterolaemia, raised alanine aminotransferase (ALT) and alkaline phosphatase (ALP), eosinopaenia, lymphopaenia and mild monocytosis. Hyperadrenocorticism was confirmed and treated but the dog deteriorated four months later and was euthanised. Two of the main macroscopic lesions are outlined below in Figs 11.3 and 11.4.

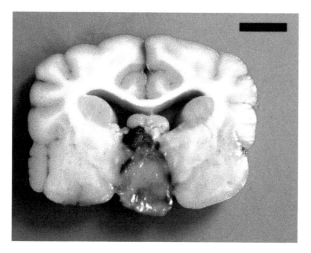

Fig. 11.3 **Bar = 1 cm.**

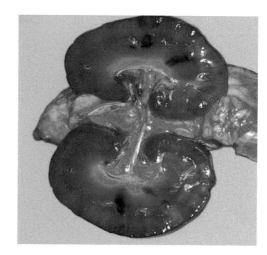

Fig. 11.4

## Questions

1. Describe any abnormalities.
2. Provide a diagnosis.
3. How would you link the lesions in Figs 11.3 and 11.4?

# END4

## Topics

Lesion recognition

Generation of pathological differential diagnoses lists

## History

A 20Y old, male neutered domestic short-haired cat was euthanised following a history of chronic renal disease. The thyroid and external parathyroid glands from this cat are shown in Fig. 11.5.

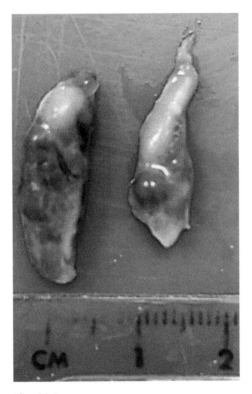

Fig. 11.5

## Questions

1. Describe any abnormalities.
2. Provide a diagnosis.
3. Explain the significance of these findings.

# END5

## Topic

**Lesion recognition**

## History

A 13Y old, male neutered Dalmatian was euthanised due to a deteriorating clinical condition. There was a history of an adrenal carcinoma, removed 6 months previously. Figs 11.6 and 11.7 depict two of the most pertinent gross lesions at the time of necropsy (note the prior surgical site is on the lower left area of image 1).

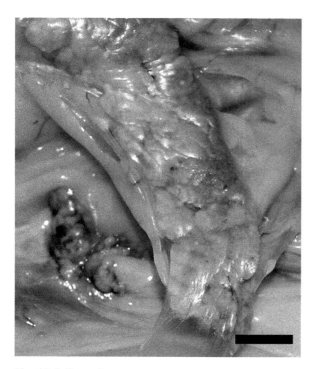

Fig. 11.6 **Bar = 1 cm.**

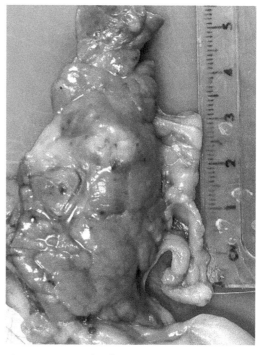

Fig. 11.7 **Formalin-fixed.**

## Questions

1. Describe any abnormalities in Figs 11.6 and 11.7.
2. Provide a diagnosis.
3. What is the significance of the pancreatic findings?

# END1 answers

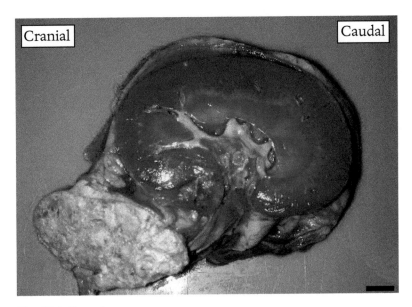

Fig. 11.1 Bar = 1 cm.

## 1. Describe any abnormalities

At the cranial pole of the kidney, in the region of the adrenal gland, there is a well-demarcated ovoid, tan/yellow, solid mass, measuring approximately 5 cm × 3 cm × 2 cm. The renal cortex contains a 1 mm diameter yellow nodule and the renal pelvis is mildly dilated, resulting in exposure of the inner renal calyces.

## 2. Provide a diagnosis

This is an adrenocortical adenocarcinoma. The mass is in the region of the adrenal gland, but it has completely obliterated the gland and is quite large, features that would support malignancy. A further sentinel of malignancy is the 1 mm nodule in the renal cortex – this is a metastatic deposit. The tan/yellow colour of these tumours is typical of adrenocortical neoplasia and is due to the high levels of cholesterol (required to make steroid hormones). Adrenocortical adenomas occur more frequently than adrenocortical adenocarcinomas; both are more likely to occur in old dogs and may be bilateral. The mild dilation of the renal pelvis is consistent with mild hydronephrosis, possibly secondary to obstruction of the ureter in this case.

## 3. Why might there be cortical atrophy of the contralateral adrenal gland?

If the tumour was functional, i.e. producing cortisol, then this would result in negative feedback to the pituitary gland, reducing production of adrenocorticotrophic hormone (ACTH). The lack of ACTH stimulation to both glands would lead to cortical atrophy in the non-neoplastic adrenal gland (and also in the gland with the neoplasm if we could see pre-existing cortex).

# END2 answers

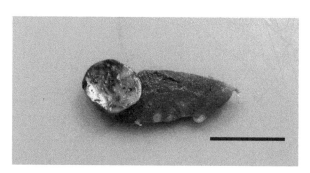

Fig. 11.2 **Formalin-fixed.**

## 1.    Describe any abnormalities

The image illustrates the thyroid and parathyroid glands. In the region of the parathyroid gland there is a well-demarcated, compressive, white mass with black mottling, measuring approximately 0.7 cm diameter. This is a great example of a benign neoplasm – well-defined, solitary, compressive, expansile*.

*Expansile: 'relating to or capable of expansion'. This is a dictionary definition, but it does not quite satisfy in pathology terms. Instead, imagine a balloon being inflated against something soft – it will just gently displace adjacent soft structures rather than invade or destroy them – that is generally how a benign tumour grows.

## 2.    Provide a diagnosis

Parathyroid adenoma.

## 3.    This is an example of primary hyperparathyroidism. Outline (a) the normal function of the parathyroid gland and (b) the pathogenesis of primary hyperparathyroidism and how it impacts on pathological features of this case.

a. In normal circumstances, parathyroid hormone (PTH) is produced as a response to reduced serum calcium. PTH (indirectly) influences osteoclasts to resorb or 'mine' calcium from the bone, increasing circulating calcium. Calcium must be maintained within a very narrow range, so this titration is an ongoing, finely balanced process. When calcium levels become too high, calcitonin, produced by C-cells in the thyroid gland, prevents osteoclasts from removing calcium from the bone and serum calcium levels drop again.

b. In primary hyperparathyroidism, the neoplastic parathyroid gland escapes normal regulatory control and turns 'rogue'. It continues to produce parathyroid hormone in the face of elevated calcium levels (normally, parathyroid hormone would decrease as calcium levels increase). As it is neoplastic, the enlarged parathyroid gland is usually **unilateral** (as in this case). The continually elevated PTH can potentially lead to many abnormalities, including soft tissue mineralisation (the chalky plaques in this case). In cases that are more prolonged there is excessive resorption of bone with cortical thinning, weakness, fractures and lameness. 'Rubber jaw' (fibrous osteodystrophy) is a well described lesion in which bone is lost due to excessive resorption and replaced by fibrous connective tissue; it is more commonly seen with secondary hyperparathyroidism.[1] This tends to occur in the flat bones of the skull and may lead to loosening of teeth. There may also be tubular mineralisation in the kidneys – nephrocalcinosis – due to increased urinary excretion of calcium (and phosphorus).

> **TIP**
>
> Whenever you need to sample a paired endocrine organ, **ALWAYS** take both glands, i.e. they should be treated as a single organ.
>
> For example, it may be difficult to interpret the possible pathogenesis of adrenal cortical atrophy without evaluation of the other adrenal gland. It is also wise to examine the pituitary gland in case there is a lesion there too.

## Reference

1    Rosol, T. J., & Meuten, D. J. (2016). Tumors of the endocrine glands. . In D. J. Meuten (Ed.) *Tumors in domestic animals* (5th ed) (pp. 766–833). Wiley.

# END3 answers

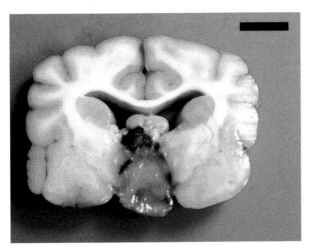

Fig. 11.3  Bar = 1 cm.

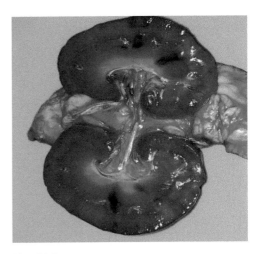

Fig. 11.4

## 1.    Describe any abnormalities

Fig. 11.3 illustrates an ill-defined mass obliterating the pituitary gland (the section is taken at the level of the basal nuclei). The mass is grey and measures approximately 1 cm diameter. It is partially surrounded by multifocal to coalescing, dark orange/brown lesions that measure up to approximately 3 mm diameter (haemorrhage).

Fig. 11.4 depicts a kidney sectioned longitudinally. The parenchyma contains multiple dark red, well-demarcated, wedge-shaped lesions that fan from the medulla towards the cortex and measure up to ~ 2 cm × 3 cm.

## 2.    Provide a diagnosis

There are two diagnoses for this case:

a.    pituitary carcinoma with haemorrhage (Fig. 11.3)
b.    multiple acute renal infarcts (Fig. 11.4).

## 3.    How would you link the lesions in Figs 11.3 and 11.4?

Some pituitary tumours can be functional, i.e. they produce excess adrenocorticotrophic hormone (ACTH). Excess ACTH stimulates increased cortisol production by the adrenal glands and the excess cortisol leads to various clinical effects, such as PU/PD, muscle wastage, 'pot belly', alopecia and lethargy. Cortisol can also favour a pro-coagulant state, leading to increased thrombosis and providing an explanation for the renal infarcts in this case (Fig. 11.4).

# END4 answers

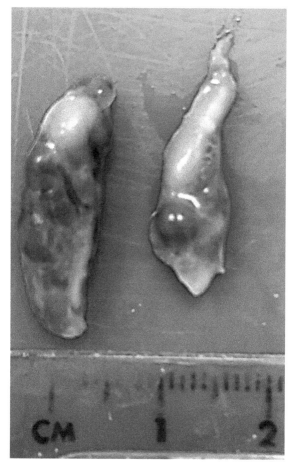

Fig. 11.5

## 1. Describe any abnormalities

The thyroid glands are asymmetrical: the smaller thyroid gland (right of the image) has a focal, smooth, brown, nodular area measuring approximately 5 mm diameter; the left thyroid gland is larger with an irregular/nodular surface. Bilaterally the external parathyroid glands are enlarged (up to 10 mm diameter on the left).

## 2. Provide a diagnosis

a. Moderate (left) to mild (right) multinodular hyperplasia – thyroid glands.

b. Moderate, bilateral parathyroid gland hyperplasia – parathyroid glands.

## 3. Explain the significance of these findings

The nodular changes within the thyroid glands are most consistent with multinodular hyperplasia, which is a common, age-related finding in older cats, also perhaps more historically known as adenomatous hyperplasia. As multinodular hyperplasia is often functional in cats (i.e.

associated with hyperthyroidism due to excessive production of $T_4$ [thyroxine] and $T_3$ [triiodothyronine]), it may result in hypertension and concentric hypertrophy of the left ventricle and so the heart should be carefully examined in this animal.

Given the clinical history of chronic renal disease, the enlarged parathyroid glands are likely secondary to renal secondary hyperparathyroidism, which has been reported to occur less commonly in cats than dogs.[1] Other non-renal lesions of uraemia may include dehydration, anaemia, ulcerative glossitis and stomatitis, pulmonary oedema, pulmonary and intercostal (subpleural) mineralisation, fibrinous pericarditis (also reportedly more common in dogs) and uraemic gastritis.[1]

## Reference

1 Ambrosio, M. B., Hennig, M. M., Nascimento, H. H. L., Santos, A. D., Flores, M. M., Fighera, R. A., Irigoyen, L. F., & Kommers, G. D. (2020). Non-renal lesions of uraemia in domestic cats. *Journal of Comparative Pathology, 180*, 105–114. https://doi.org/10.1016/j.jcpa.2020.09.004

# END5 answers

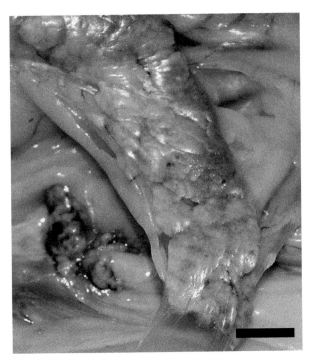

Fig. 11.6 **Bar = 1 cm.**

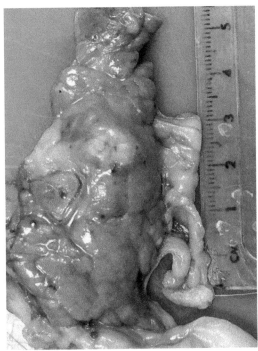

Fig. 11.7 **Formalin-fixed.**

## 1. Describe any abnormalities in Figs 11.6 and 11.7

In Fig 11.6, in the region of the prior surgery (adrenal gland bed), there is a very irregular, micronodular, pink mass measuring ~2 cm × 1.5 cm. Within the pancreas, there are scattered, 2–4 mm diameter, off-white foci. In Fig. 11.7, some of these small foci are visible, with a larger, 1 cm diameter, off-white and slightly centrally depressed (umbilicated) nodule also present.

## 2. Provide a diagnosis

There are three diagnoses:

a. recurrence of adrenal carcinoma
b. pancreatic exocrine nodular hyperplasia
c. pancreatic neoplasia.

## 3. What is the significance of the pancreatic findings?

The smaller nodules in the pancreas (Fig. 11.6) are consistent with pancreatic exocrine nodular hyperplasia, which is a common, incidental and age-related finding in the pancreas of older dogs. The larger nodule (Fig. 11.7) may be an adenoma or adenocarcinoma of the exocrine or endocrine portions of the pancreas. Histopathology is essential for a final diagnosis (this was a pancreatic adenocarcinoma) but if there is a clinical history of hypoglycaemia in the patient, it could be an insulinoma (i.e. a tumour of the endocrine beta

cells of the pancreatic islets). See Fig. 11.7a for annotations of the lesions in Fig 11.6.

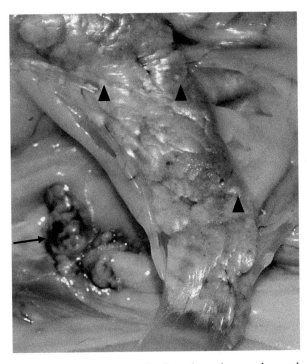

Fig. 11.7a **Recurrence of adrenal carcinoma (arrow) and foci of pancreatic exocrine nodular hyperplasia (arrowheads).**

# Complex cases

**12**

# COMPLEX1

Topics

Practical technique

Lesion recognition

Approach to difficult cases

## History

There was very little history available for this adult female domestic shorthair cat that was found dead in a garden. Animal cruelty prevention officers submitted it to a local veterinary practice for necropsy (Fig 12.1).

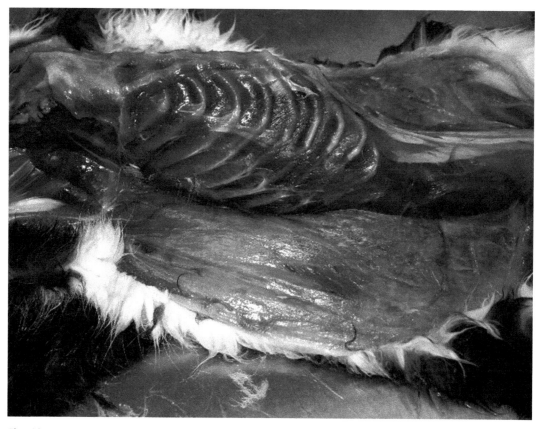

Fig. 12.1

## Questions

1. Describe any abnormalities.
2. Provide a diagnosis.
3. What issues would you consider if you were the veterinary surgeon in charge of the case?

# COMPLEX2

## Topics

Approach to difficult cases

Generation of pathological differential diagnoses lists

Integration of pathological findings with clinical aspects

## History

A 6Y old, male intact German Shepherd Dog was found dead after a brief period of generalised weakness. The main necropsy findings are illustrated in Fig. 12.2.

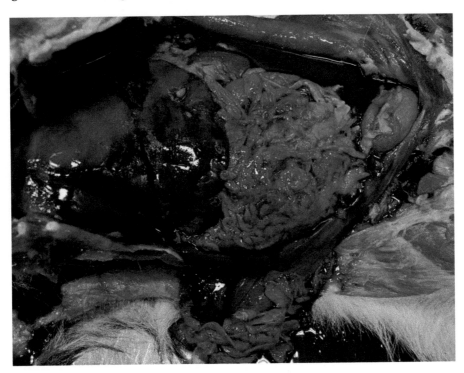

Fig. 12.2

## Questions

1. Describe any abnormalities.
2. Provide a diagnosis.
3. Provide some differentials for this pathological presentation. **Briefly** outline some specific sampling approaches in this case.

# COMPLEX3

## Topics

Approach to difficult cases

Common artefacts and pitfalls

## History

A 4Y old, female neutered domestic longhair cat died during a routine dental procedure. The cat was necropsied and Figs 12.3 and 12.4 are of the thoracic and abdominal cavities, respectively.

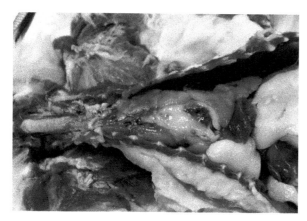

Fig. 12.3

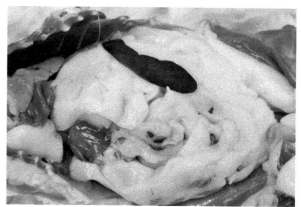

Fig. 12.4

## Questions

1. Describe any abnormalities.
2. Provide a diagnosis.
3. Briefly outline your next steps.

# COMPLEX1 answers

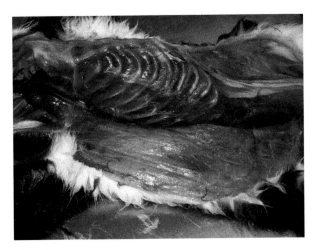

Fig. 12.1

## 1.   Describe any abnormalities

There is no subcutaneous body fat and there is a loss of general muscle mass. Tissues also appear a little tacky, though this is difficult to evaluate from the image alone.

## 2.   Provide a diagnosis

Emaciation and diffuse muscle atrophy.

A tacky texture in soft tissues can be an indicator of dehydration, albeit a subjective one (if the eyes have sunk into their orbits then this provides further supportive evidence of dehydration).

## 3.   What issues would you consider if you were the veterinary surgeon in charge of the case?

We deliberately gave very little history in this case to try to stimulate consideration of multiple possibilities. Questions that may be raised at this stage are: (a) Was this someone's pet cat or was it a stray? (b) Was it intentionally abused/starved? (c) Did it have an underlying health condition that weakened it, perhaps leading to a road traffic accident (RTA)?

The most striking finding in the necropsy thus far (the body is yet to be opened) is emaciation, which means complete loss of body fat. In this case there is also generalised loss of muscle mass (muscle atrophy). This combination may be due to prolonged malnutrition/starvation or cachexia secondary to an underlying disease condition, particularly malignant neoplasia. There was also no internal body fat; during necropsy, good places to look are around the heart, around the kidneys and in the bone marrow. Serous atrophy of fat (where the fat becomes clear and gelatinous due to loss of lipids), particularly in the bone marrow, is a reliable signal that an animal has been mal-

nourished for some time (see Fig. 12.1a below). In such cases, it is important to rule out underlying disease, so a complete necropsy must be performed.

Other pertinent aspects of this type of necropsy are outlined below.

1.   Weigh the animal (which should be a part of any necropsy, where feasible).
2.   Scan the body for an identity chip and record any other identifiers, such as a tattoo.
3.   Examine the entire alimentary system (oral cavity/teeth, gastrointestinal tract) and record (a) the presence and quantity of ingesta in the stomach; (b) the presence of any intestinal content, especially formed faeces in the rectum; (c) the presence or absence of endoparasites.
4.   Methodically examine and dissect **ALL** organs (including brain, endocrine organs and joints), even if the body is very autolysed.
5.   Collect a range of samples for histopathology in case further investigation is required. In this type of case, it would also be prudent to collect fresh samples from major organs (liver, kidney, stomach content; heart blood; urine; fat; brain) should toxicology become necessary. Such samples can be frozen indefinitely at −20°C. This is not a step you would necessarily include for non-forensic necropsies.
6.   If you need to culture any organs, this should be done at the time of the necropsy – avoid freezing samples destined for culture as freezing often affects the viability of organisms. Equally, if the body has already been frozen, culture is probably going to be unrewarding.
7.   Bearing in mind the cat may have suffered trauma, the limb bones, skull, ribs, spinal column and pelvis should be assessed for a fracture (soft tissue haemorrhage around the fracture is usually evident but palpation may also be required). A cat's claws are a good place to look for evidence of trauma since they are often shredded and broken, but another helpful approach is to skin the body at the end of the necropsy, since lesions such as bruising or puncture wounds may be otherwise overlooked as they are difficult to see due to the hair coat. You might even consider radiography if available. This can be helpful to assess fractured bones but also provides internal evidence of gunshot pellets.
8.   Most importantly, document all findings in writing and consider taking supportive photographs.

Before beginning the necropsy, you should consider submitting cases like this to a veterinary pathologist, especially if the case is of interest to the authorities and/or the legal system (i.e. it becomes a forensic case). Even if not of forensic interest at the start, it may become so later. If you are not in a position to do this (e.g. for geographical reasons), then it would be advisable to at least discuss handling of the case before and after with a veterinary pathologist. If there is no other option, cases like this can be frozen until such time as transport to a pathologist becomes practical. But freezing should be a last resort!

Also bear in mind that, depending on jurisdiction in your part of the country, you may need to consider having corroboration of your findings by another veterinary professional, which can include a veterinary nurse or, depending on work location, necropsy room technical staff.

Also see: Chapter 1, Approach to forensic necropsy cases; Chapter 1, Necropsy sampling guidelines.

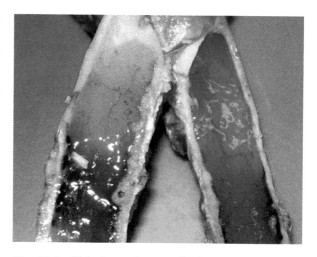

Fig. 12.1a This femur is actually from an emaciated sheep but it is a good example of the distinctive gross appearance of serous atrophy of fat in the marrow space, an appearance which is not species specific. The normal fat has been replaced by gelatinous, transparent, amber material.

# COMPLEX2 answers

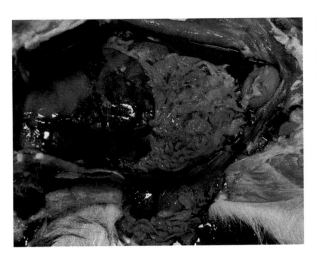

Fig. 12.2

## 1.  Describe any abnormalities

The abdominal cavity contains a large amount of free, unclotted blood. The volume measured at time of necropsy was 700 ml and the thoracic cavity contained 465 ml of blood. (The liver discolouration is most likely due to autolysis and the blood in the abdomen will have resulted in the discolouration of the mesenteric fat.)

## 2.  Provide a diagnosis

Marked haemoabdomen.

## 3.  Provide some differentials for this pathological presentation. **Briefly** outline some specific sampling approaches in this case.

Differentials: Broad causes of haemorrhage are (a) trauma (b) coagulopathy (c) vascular disease.

It is unlikely that vascular disease would or could lead to this type and degree of haemorrhage, so (a) and (b) are much more likely. Trauma should be excluded as far as possible by skinning the body to look for evidence of external bruising, assessing visceral organs for fractures/tears, and checking for bone fractures (e.g. pelvis, ribs, skull, spinal column). Also, ensure that you check major vessels and organs for any rupture sites. Further differentials for a coagulopathy are:

1. disseminated intravascular coagulopathy (DIC)
2. thrombocytopaenia* or abnormal platelet function

3. deficiency of clotting factors (DIC, toxin exposure [e.g. dicoumarol], chronic liver disease, vitamin K deficiency, inherited clotting factor deficiency although this is unlikely in an older dog with no prior history of haemorrhage).

Sample collection in this case mainly focuses on the causes of a coagulopathy. Bone marrow is important to collect but it does autolyse quickly so should be sampled as soon after death as possible. Liver is obvious but major visceral organs should be collected in any sudden death, including lungs, heart and kidneys. These samples are fixed for histopathology but a fresh panel of organs suitable for toxicology is also vital (standard panel: stomach contents, liver, kidney, blood† and urine if present – fat, brain and lung are also worth collecting to allow for a wider panel of testing if required later). Tissues destined for toxicology can be frozen without adversely affecting testing.

## Text notes

* Thrombocytopaenia may be caused by the following:

1. decreased production:
    a. targeted suppression or platelets by the immune system (immune-mediated destruction of megakaryocytes) or drugs
    b. general suppression of haematopoiesis in the marrow by neoplasia; fibrosis; radiation; infection; chemicals
2. increased destruction or consumption: immune mediated; DIC (e.g. due to sepsis, neoplasia, organ failure, pancreatitis or severe inflammation)
3. a change in distribution: sequestration in a diseased spleen.

† Any free body cavity blood or fluid will suffice, or blood collected from the chambers of the heart, clotted or unclotted.

> TIP
>
> Loss of this volume of blood in a German Shepherd Dog could easily cause hypovolaemic shock and death.
> - A large male GSD might weigh up to 40 kg.
> - Blood accounts for 7% of bodyweight = 2.8 l.
> - Loss of 40% of blood volume will generally lead to death through hypovolaemia = 1.12 l.
> - This dog lost 1.165 l.

# COMPLEX3 answers

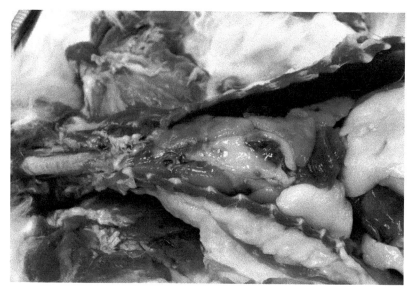

Fig. 12.3

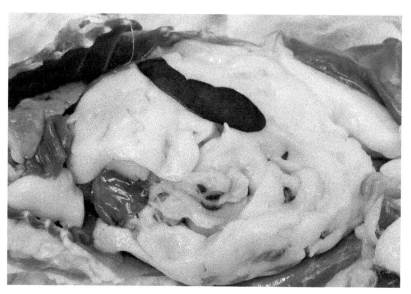

Fig. 12.4

## 1.   Describe any abnormalities

There are none. The images depict grossly normal thoracic and abdominal cavities. There is above average internal fat which obscures the gastrointestinal tract, liver, pancreas and urinary tract but they were also grossly normal. The lungs are salmon pink with slight apical overinflation (postmortem change in this case). The yellow discolouration of the fat is a good example of bile imbibition, a postmortem change. There is no evidence of fat necrosis (which could indicate pancreatitis), peritonitis, haemorrhage or trauma. The spleen is grossly normal. The images also show that the body was in very good postmortem condition with little evidence of autolysis.

## 2.   Provide a diagnosis

In such a case, the diagnosis would be 'Open' or 'Inconclusive'.

## 3.   Briefly outline your next steps

Keep going! You have opened it up now and it is too late to seek external antemortem advice, other than over the telephone (which is still worth pursuing). Complete a full and thorough examination, including removal and evaluation of the brain, with supportive notes *and photographs*. Take representative samples of all visceral organs and the gastrointestinal tract for histopathology, as well as any grossly visible lesions. Pay close attention to the cardiovascular and respiratory systems. Ideally, the brain and opened heart should be fixed in their entirety and retained for histopathology. Other tissues of potential value for histopathology include skeletal muscle, diaphragm, endocrine glands (take both if paired) bone marrow (if fresh enough), thymus (if present), skin, peripheral nerve(s) and multiple lymph nodes. If a cause of death is not immediately obvious macroscopically, then histological evaluation of a range of tissues may help to identify underlying pre-existing disease, which may have weakened the cat and predisposed it to death under anaesthetic (e.g. sepsis, myocarditis, pneumonia, neoplasia, anaemia). Retain samples of frozen organs as back up (liver, kidney, blood, stomach contents and urine as a minimum). Have a qualified colleague review your findings.

> Given this death is anaesthetic-associated, you should strongly consider referring the necropsy to an independent veterinary pathologist prior to any other actions.

## Comment

Anaesthetic-associated deaths are infrequent in cats, but more common than in dogs and humans. In our experience, a macroscopic cause is often not found. This is corroborated by the literature, though there is variation in the reported rate of anaesthetic-associated deaths where no cause is apparent (36–63%).[1,2] Where gross findings are evident, they tend to involve the heart and/or lungs, although systemic disease (notably systemic infections) is also reported, hence the need to examine tissues histologically.

Lack of a defined cause at necropsy does not automatically imply that the anaesthetic caused death. There are other possible causes that may be responsible in the absence of lesions. Gerdin et al.[2] summarise a few potential complications arising from the anaesthetic procedure that cannot be confirmed by necropsy. They include upper airway occlusion by the soft palate or incorrect endotracheal tube placement; respiratory acidosis secondary to hypoventilation; and cardiac conduction abnormalities (e.g. dysrhythmia). Over the years we have occasionally been asked by vets or clients if we can test anaesthetic levels using toxicology, but such techniques are currently not viable in veterinary medicine and would be impossible to validate given the many factors that may influence anaesthetic levels in the animal's body at any one time.

## References

1  DeLay, J. (2016). Perianesthetic mortality in domestic animals: A retrospective study of postmortem lesions and review of autopsy procedures. *Veterinary Pathology*, *53*(5), 1078–1086. https://doi.org/10.1177/0300985816655853

2  Gerdin, J. A., Slater, M. R., Makolinski, K. V., Looney, A. L., Appel, L. D., Martin, N. M., & McDonough, S. P. (2011). Postmortem findings in 54 cases of anesthetic associated death in cats from two spay-neuter programs in New York State. *Journal of Feline Medicine and Surgery*, *13*(12), 959–966. https://doi.org/10.1016/j.jfms.2011.07.021